Medicines

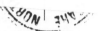

The *Essential Clinical Skills for Nurses* series focuses on key clinical skills for nurses and other health professionals. These concise, accessible books assume no prior knowledge and focus on core clinical skills, clearly presenting common clinical procedures and their rationale, together with the essential background theory. Their user-friendly format makes them an indispensable guide to clinical practice for all nurses, especially to student nurses and newly qualified staff.

Other titles in the *Essential Clinical Skills for Nurses* series:

Medicines Management

A Guide for Nurses

Edited by

Philip Jevon
RN, BSc(Hons), PGCE
Resuscitation Officer/Clinical Skills Lead
Manor Hospital
Walsall, UK
Honorary Clinical Lecturer
University of Birmingham, UK

Elizabeth Payne
BSc(Hons) in Pharmacy, MSc in Clinical Pharmacy,
MRPharmS
Deputy Director of Pharmacy, Education,
Training and Staff Performance
Manor Hospital
Walsall, UK

Dan Higgins
RGN, ENB 100, ENB 998
Senior Charge Nurse Critical Care
University Hospitals Birmingham NHS Foundation Trust
Consultant/Honorary Lecturer Resuscitation Services UK
Visiting Clinical Lecturer
University of Birmingham, UK

Ruth Endacott
RN, DipN(Lond), MA, PhD
Professor of Clinical Nursing
University of Plymouth, UK and La Trobe University, Australia

⟨W⟩ WILEY-BLACKWELL

A John Wiley & Sons, Ltd., Publication

This edition first published 2010
© 2010 by Blackwell Publishing Ltd

Blackwell Publishing was acquired by John Wiley & Sons in February 2007. Blackwell's publishing programme has been merged with Wiley's global Scientific, Technical, and Medical business to form Wiley-Blackwell.

Registered office
John Wiley & Sons Ltd, The Atrium, Southern Gate, Chichester, West Sussex, PO19 8SQ, United Kingdom

Editorial offices
9600 Garsington Road, Oxford, OX4 2DQ, United Kingdom
2121 State Avenue, Ames, Iowa 50014-8300, USA

For details of our global editorial offices, for customer services and for information about how to apply for permission to reuse the copyright material in this book please see our website at www.wiley.com/wiley-blackwell.

Library of Congress Cataloging-in-Publication Data

Medicines management : a guide for nurses / edited by Philip Jevon . . . [et al.].
p. ; cm. – (Essential clinical skills for nurses)
Includes bibliographical references and index.
ISBN 978-1-4051-8163-1 (pbk. : alk. paper) 1. Drugs–Administration–Handbooks, manuals, etc. 2. Nursing–Handbooks, manuals, etc. 3. Therapeutics–Handbooks, manuals, etc. I. Jevon, Philip. II. Series: Essential clinical skills for nurses.
[DNLM: 1. Drug Therapy–nursing–Great Britain. 2. Drug Monitoring–nursing–Great Britain. 3. Medication Errors–prevention & control–Great Britain. 4. Nurse's Role–Great Britain. 5. Prescriptions–nursing–Great Britain. WY 100 M4899 2010]
RM125.M37 2010
615'.1068–dc22
2009037332

A catalogue record for this book is available from the British Library.

Set in 9 on 11 pt Palatino by Toppan Best-set Premedia Limited
Printed and bound in Malaysia by KHL Printing Co Sdn Bhd

1 2010

Contents

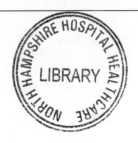

Contents

Foreword

Effective and safe medicines management is a key responsibility for all nurses and midwives. The pace of change in this area in recent years has been breathtaking, with the ever-increasing range and complexity of medicines themselves, and the developments in regulation and legislation relating to prescribing and administration. Nurses and midwives have a professional responsibility to keep up-to-date with new developments, guidelines and regulations, and with all aspects of patient safety.

This book details the key components of medicines management from basic pharmacology and principles of safe administration to nurse prescribing. The multi-disciplinary authorship ensures that it is a well balanced, helpful and reliable resource. I congratulate the authors on their achievement.

I would recommend this book for pre-registration and post-registration nurses and midwives. Nurse tutors would also find it helpful and informative and it will be useful for other healthcare professionals concerned with medicines management.

Jane Hare BPharm, MRPharmS
Director of Pharmacy, Walsall Hospitals NHS Trust

Contributors List

Matthew Aldridge RN, RNT, MA(Ed), BSc(Hons), FHEA
Senior Lecturer in Clinical Skills, Faculty of Health, Birmingham
City University, UK

Ruth Endacott RN, DipN(Lond), MA, PhD
Professor of Clinical Nursing at the University of Plymouth, UK
and La Trobe University, Australia

Brian Gammon BA, MMedSc, RN, PhD
Clinical Trials Practitioner, Sandwell and West Birmingham
Hospitals NHS Trust, Birmingham, UK

Richard Griffith LLM, BN, DipN, PgdL, RMN, Cert Ed, RNT
Lecturer in Health Law, School of Health Science, Swansea
University, UK

Dan Higgins RGN, ENB 100, ENB 998
Senior Charge Nurse Critical Care, University Hospitals
Birmingham NHS Foundation Trust and Consultant/Honorary
Lecturer Resuscitation Services UK and Visiting Clinical Lecturer,
University of Birmingham, UK

Janet Hunter MA, BSc(Hons)
RN Senior Lecturer in Adult Nursing, School of Community and
Health Sciences, West Smithfield, City University London, UK

**Elizabeth Payne BSc(Hons) in Pharmacy, MSc in Clinical
Pharmacy, MRPharmS**
Deputy Director of Pharmacy, Education, Training and Staff
Performance, Manor Hospital, Walsall, UK

Kate Roland MPharm, PgD Pharm Prac, MRPharm S
Domiciliary Pharmacist, Devon PCT and Devon County Council, UK

Gareth Walters BSc(Hons), MBChB, MRCP(UK), MRCP(London), AHEA, MInstLM, LCGI
Specialist Registrar in Respiratory and General Medicine, West Midlands Rotation and Honorary Clinical Lecturer, University of Birmingham, UK

Introduction to Medicines Management

1

Ruth Endacott

INTRODUCTION

The term 'medicines management' has become increasingly popular over the last 10 years, but what exactly does it mean? The NHS National Prescribing Centre (NPC) provides the following definition:

> *A system of processes and behaviours that determines how medicines are used by patients and by the NHS.*

> (NPC, 2001, p. 5)

This encompasses all activities necessary to select, purchase, deliver, prescribe, administer, store and review medication (Audit Commission, 2001). Pharmacies have provided specific components of medicines management services for many years. However, the responsibility for medicines management services is not only held by pharmacists but also shared with other healthcare professionals and the patients themselves.

So it is true to say that medicines management is not a new concept but an evolving concept, emphasising patient-focused care and services that help deliver that care.

LEARNING OUTCOMES

At the end of this chapter, the reader will be able to:

❏ Discuss the importance of medicines management.
❏ Discuss the context of medicines management in the UK.
❏ List the elements of medicines management.
❏ Outline medicines management and health service governance procedures.
❏ Discuss the impact of medicines management on patient safety.

❑ List the success factors for improving medicines management.

IMPORTANCE OF MEDICINES MANAGEMENT

Medication is by far the most common form of medical intervention, and at least 20% of Primary Care Trust (PCT) funds are spent in this area (NPC, 2001). Most patients are given medication on discharge from hospital, and up to 40% of nurses' time is spent administering medications (Audit Commission, 2001). Four out of five people over 75 years take a prescription medicine, and 36% are taking four or more [Department of Health (DH), 2001].

The prime driver for medicines management is to enhance the overall standard of patient care and to ensure safe and effective use of medicines. Obviously, this is very good news for the patient, but additional improved treatment outcomes can have a knock-on effect in other areas of the health service. The English National Service Framework (NSF) for older people states that medicines are implicated in 5–17% of hospital admissions in this patient group, and whilst in hospital 6–17% of older people experience adverse reactions to medicines (DH, 2001). More recently, a review of patients readmitted to hospital in this age group identified that 38% of readmissions were related to medications (Witherington *et al.*, 2008). Many of these incidents could be avoided if better medicines management systems were in place.

Evidence on medicine taking indicates that 50% of people with chronic conditions may not be taking medicines as intended (DH, 2001). This includes essential medicines for life-threatening conditions such as anti-hypertensive treatment for high blood pressures and anti-rejection treatment post organ transplantation.

Medicines management is also essential to control the NHS drugs bill. New drugs and formulations, changes in demographics and government policies, along with increased patient expectations have caused the drugs bill to rise year on year. If medicines are managed properly, for instance through rational prescribing and effective waste control measures, the NHS can save money, which can then be used more effectively on other treatments. Integrated processes for medicines management also enable local policies to be developed for the introduction of high-cost drugs, for which there is no National Institute for Clinical Excellence (NICE) guidance. The ongoing cost implications of these medications have an impact across health services, hence policies need to be developed in consultation with a range of stakeholders.

A DH review of adverse events (*An Organisation with a Memory*) identified that around 10 000 NHS hospital patients a year experience adverse effects related to medicines and 20% of all clinical negligence litigation relates to hospital medication errors (DH, 2000). The Audit Commission (2001) identified that medication errors cost the NHS £500m each year and, more importantly, medication errors are responsible for about 20% of the deaths that are due to adverse events in hospital.

THE CONTEXT OF MEDICINES MANAGEMENT IN THE UK

National context

The modernisation programme for the NHS includes an important agenda to improve medicines management. There are a number of key documents (Appendix 1.1) that embrace medicines management and provide broad objectives to improve the use of medicines within the NHS.

The services provided by the NHS are changing to meet national expectations and the expectations of service users and carers. Changes in medicines management is a key part of this process.

Medicines management makes a significant contribution to the Care Quality Commission Annual Health Check and Standards for Better Health (for more information, see www.cqc.org.uk/publications.cfm?fde_id=679, accessed 4 November 2009). It features in several domains but largely within the safety domain to 'keep patients, staff and visitors safe by having systems to ensure that medicines are handled safely and securely'.

Standards for medicines management are also included in the primary care Quality Outcomes Framework (QOF) and form part of the General Medical Services contract (www.bma.org.uk/employmentandcontracts/independent_contractors/quality_outcomes_framework/focusQOF0308.jsp, accessed 22 June 2009).

Indicator points for medicines management, against which funding is provided to GP practices, include the following:

- The practice possesses the equipment and in-date emergency drugs to treat anaphylaxis.
- There is a system for checking the expiry dates of emergency drugs on at least an annual basis.
- The number of hours from requesting a prescription to availability for collection by the patient is 72 hours or less (excluding weekends and bank/local holidays).
- A medication review is recorded in the notes in the preceding 15 months for all patients being prescribed four or more repeat medicines.

National initiatives have been translated into specific benchmarks in many areas, see, for example, the benchmarking policy for medicines management at Eastern and Coastal Kent PCT at www.eastkentcoastalpct.nhs.uk/search/?q=medicines+management+benchmarking+policy).

Local context

The current focus for medicines management within an NHS Trust is the Drug and Therapeutics Committee. This committee meets every month and is chaired by a consultant biochemist who works closely with the Director of Pharmacy to plan the agenda. The committee is accountable to the Clinical Governance Committee and via the Medical Director to the Trust Board. Information and decisions from the committee are communicated via the Medicines Information Bulletin and EnLine.

A Medication Safety Group, made up of doctors, pharmacists and nurses from across the Trust, examines clinical incidents involving medication and makes recommendations to reduce the frequency of these incidents.

The Chief Pharmacist sits on the Clinical Effectiveness Subgroup to ensure that medicines-related aspects of NICE guidance are implemented and on the Executive Board to ensure that medicines and their use are accounted for when Trust-wide decisions are made. The Chief Pharmacist and Chair of the Drug and Therapeutics Committee also represent the Trust on a Countywide Prescribing Group with a wider health community role.

ELEMENTS OF MEDICINES MANAGEMENT

Medicines management includes the selection, procurement, delivery, prescription, dispensing and administration of medicines. The NPC (2008) has developed a flowchart to illustrate how these processes intersect (see Figure 1.1).

Selection and procurement

Decisions about which drugs will be available for clinicians to prescribe and where the drugs will be purchased are taken at Trust level. The medicines management pathway (Figure 1.1) is one tool that is used by commissioners of health services to assess the prescribing and medicines implications of a new clinical pathway (for example, an NSF or a new pathway for managing a particular disease). The potential impact of raising public health awareness (for example, sexual health and smoking cessation campaigns) on prescribing practices is also considered as part of an integrated medicines management system.

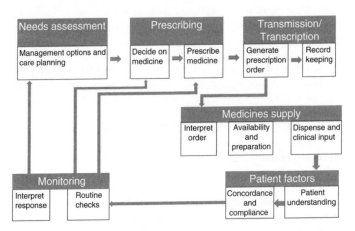

Fig 1.1 Medicines management pathway. From 'Moving towards personalising medicines management: improving outcomes for people through the safe and effective use of medicines' (April 2008). Copyright National Prescribing Centre, reproduced by permission.

Handling

Medicines must be stored according to specific instructions; details for all medications can be found in the electronic Medicines Compendium (see www.emc.medicines.org.uk), including summaries of product characteristics (SPCs) and patient information leaflets. SPCs are written and updated by pharmaceutical companies, in accordance with a mandatory proforma, and are approved by the UK or European medicines licensing agency.

Prescription

Regular review of prescribing practices is recommended as good practice and is rewarded as part of the QOF funding for patients receiving repeat prescriptions. To take an example from mental health, such a repeat prescribing review would include the following questions in discussion with the service user:

- Are the medicines making a positive difference? Is the service user feeling better?
- What side effects are being experienced?
- What are the options for addressing these?
- What healthy living options, such as diet, physical activity, alcohol reduction and smoking cessation, might be appropriate?
- Is the service user having problems remembering to take the medication? If so, what 'concordance' support can be arranged, such as the use of monitored dosage systems in the form of blister packs, medication reminder charts or tablet boxes showing days of the week and times of day?

(NIHME National Workforce Programme, 2008)

Administration

An integrated approach to medicines management provides greater opportunity to identify and manage problems related to medication administration. For example, regular review of drug incidents highlights particular ward environments or times of day when medication administration is more problematic. The development of integrated electronic systems for medication management, including medication administration, is discussed in Chapter 5.

MEDICINES MANAGEMENT AND HEALTH SERVICE GOVERNANCE PROCEDURES

The growing complexity and cost of medicines have led to the recognition that medicines management is a crucial aspect of clinical and financial governance in NHS Trusts, as highlighted in the following documents:

- *Clinical Negligence Scheme for Trusts (CNST)* (NHS Litigation Authority, 2005): Two standards relate directly to medicines management and encompass a variety of areas.
- *Building a Safer NHS for Patients – Improving Medication Safety* (DH, 2004): Medicines management systems are highlighted as the most important facility in assuring patient safety in relation to medicines. The report emphasises the controls necessary to reduce errors in prescribing, dispensing and administering medicines.
- *A Spoonful of Sugar* (Audit Commission, 2001): This report describes medicines management as 'a strategic issue fundamental to the way hospitals work, to the quality of patient care and to the delivery of the NHS Plan'. The central role of pharmacists is recognised, and Trust boards are asked to ensure adequate investment in pharmacy services.
- *An Organisation with a Memory* (DH, 2000): This document emphasises the role of medicines management in reducing risks related to the use of medicines.

THE IMPACT OF MEDICINES MANAGEMENT ON PATIENT SAFETY

As previously identified, medication errors are an important factor in adverse events in health care. There is evidence that this trend is rising (Audit Commission, 2001; NPSA, 2007), with 'severe harm' from medication reported in research studies reaching as high as 9% of hospital inpatients (NPSA, 2007, p12). It is acknowledged that reported medication incidents are the tip of the iceberg; however, in the 18 months between January 2005 and June 2006, just under 60 000 medication incidents were reported to the National Patient Safety Agency, mostly occurring in hospital (NPSA, 2007).

A number of factors have been identified that may contribute to the extent of medication incidents and errors; these are discussed in Chapter 7, along with strategies to reduce medication error.

KEY SUCCESS FACTORS FOR IMPROVING MEDICINES MANAGEMENT

The NPC has identified 10 key success factors for improving medicines management (NIMHE National Workforce Programme, 2008):

1. Involving and listening to patient and carers.
2. Clear leadership.
3. Multidisciplinary approach.
4. Medicines management objectives aligned to organisational priorities.
5. Local medicines management leader.
6. Effective communication.
7. Medicines management champions.
8. Focus on measuring outcomes, not activity.
9. Protected time.
10. Shared learning and networking.

The emphasis in these success factors is firmly on communication between patients, clinicians, pharmacists and Trust boards.

CONCLUSION

This chapter has provided an introduction to medicines management. The importance of medicines management, together with its context in the UK, has been discussed. The elements of medicines management have been listed. Medicines management and health service governance procedures have been outlined, together with their impact on patient safety. Success factors for improving medicines management have been listed.

APPENDIX 1.1 RELEVANT NATIONAL STRATEGIES AND DOCUMENTS

Department of Health (2000) The NHS Plan

Department of Health (2000) Pharmacy in the Future – Implementing the NHS Plan

Department of Health (2000) An Organisation with a Memory – Report of an expert group on learning from adverse events (including the formation of the NPSA)

Audit Commission (2001) 'A Spoonful of Sugar'

Department of Health (2001) National Service Framework for Older People. The Stationery Office, London

Department of Health (2003) Medicines Management Framework in NHS Hospitals. DH, London

Department of Health (2003) A Vision for Pharmacy in the New NHS. DH, London

Department of Health (2004) Building a Safer NHS for Patients – Improving Medication Safety. DH, London

Department of Health (2004i) National Standards, Local Action: Health and social care standards and planning framework 2005/06–2007/08. DH, London

Department of Health and Department for Education and Skills (2004) National Service Framework for Children, Young People and Maternity Services. DH, London

Healthcare Commission Assessment for Improvement. The annual health check

Measuring What Matters (2005)

REFERENCES

Audit Commission (2001) *A Spoonful of Sugar: Medicines Management in NHS Hospitals*. Audit Commission, London.

Department of Health (DH) (2000) *An Organisation with a Memory: Report of an Expert Group on Learning from Adverse Events in the NHS Chaired by the Chief Medical Officer*. The Stationery Office, London.

Department of Health (DH) (2001) *Medicines and Older People – Supplement to the National Service Framework for Older People*. The Stationery Office, London.

Department of Health (DH) (2004) *Building a Safer NHS for Patients – Improving Medication Safety*. DH, London.

National Patient Safety Agency (NPSA) (2007) *Safety in Doses: Medication Safety Incidents in the NHS*. The fourth report from the Patient Safety Observatory (PSO/4). NPSA, London.

National Prescribing Centre (NPC) (2001) *Modernising Medicines Management. A Guide to Achieving Benefits for Patients, Professionals and the NHS*. NPC, London.

National Prescribing Centre (NPC) (2008) Moving towards personalising medicines management: improving outcomes for people through the safe and effective use of medicines. Available at www.npc.co.uk/mm/publications.htm?type=:medicines [accessed on 4 November 2009].

NHS Litigation Authority (2005) *CNST General Clinical Risk Management Standards*. NHSLA, London.

NIMHE National Workforce Programme (2008) *Medicines Management: Everybody's Business*. DH, London.

Witherington EMA, Pirzada OM, Avery AJ (2008) Communication gaps and readmissions to hospital for patients aged 75 years and older: observational study. *Qual Safety Health Care* **17**(1): 71–75.

Legal Issues of Medicines Management

2

Richard Griffith

INTRODUCTION

Medicines are used for their therapeutic benefits but they also have great potential to harm those who take them. Drugs such as thalidomide [*S* v *Distillers Co. (Biochemicals)* (1970)] and Opren [*Nash* v *Eli Lilly & Co* (1993)] demonstrate the tragic consequences that may follow poor medication management and administration. The law therefore regulates the arrangements for the supply and administration of medicines to patients.

The Medicines Act 1968, section 58A, requires that medicines that represent a danger to the patient be classified as prescription only and their administration be supervised by an appropriate practitioner. Nurses who meet conditions specified in law can become appropriate practitioners (Medicines Act 1968, section 58(1)). However, unlike doctors, who prescribe from one national formulary, non-medical prescribers have up to seven different roles when prescribing or administering medicines to patients, each with its own requirements and limitations. In order to practise safely and avoid legal and professional liability, nurses must ensure that they manage medicines properly and have the proper authority to prescribe or administer.

For example, a practice nurse was cautioned by the Nursing and Nursery Council's Conduct and Competence Committee when the nurse prescribed drugs to patients without having the authority to do so. The committee stressed that whilst the role of nurses and non-medical prescribers was expanding, public protection demanded that proper medication management be practised [Nursing & Midwifery Council (NMC), 2003].

LEARNING OBJECTIVES

At the end of this chapter, the reader will be able to:

❑ Identify the spheres of accountability that regulate nursing practice.

❑ Explain the regulation of clinical trials.

❑ Discuss the legal regulation of medicines.

❑ Discuss the legal regulation of controlled drugs.

❑ Outline the civil liability of nurses when managing medicines.

❑ Discuss the issues of consent.

❑ Describe the elements of good record keeping.

SPHERES OF ACCOUNTABILITY THAT REGULATE NURSING PRACTICE

As registered practitioners, nurses are answerable for their actions to four main legal sources:

- the profession;
- the employer;
- the patient;
- society.

The profession

A nurse who is found guilty of professional misconduct is liable to removal from the professional register. The Nursing and Nursery Council has the authority to hold nurses to account through the Nursing & Midwifery Order 2001. The professional standard required of a nurse by the governing body is given in the Nursing and Nursery Council's code, standards of conduct, performance and ethics for nurses (NMC, 2008a) and in relation to medicines is further elaborated in the standards for medication management (NMC, 2008c).

It is essential that registered nurses abide by the requirements of the code and comply with the standards for medication management. A total of 214 nurses were issued with striking off orders for professional misconduct in 2007–2008. Of the allegations investigated by the Council, about 14% concerned direct contact with patients and 9.87% with maladministration of medication (NMC, 2008b).

The employer

Nurses have legally binding contracts of employment with their employers, which require, among other duties, that they obey the reasonable requests of the employer and work with due care and skill. The contract further requires that nurses are duty bound to account for their actions and to disclose any misdeeds. An employer may therefore hold an employee to account through reasonable disciplinary policies and procedures, which ultimately may lead to dismissal.

For example, a nurse was sacked by her employer and subsequently suspended by the NMC when she admitted stealing medicines from the ward (Nurse struck off for stealing medicines, 2008).

As a result of the control employers exercise over their employees, the law holds them vicariously liable for any tort committed by an employee during the course of their employment, which has the effect of indemnifying the employee against damages for harm caused to another in the course of their employment.

The patient

Patients who feel that they have been harmed by the carelessness of nurses can seek redress though the civil court system. This is a lengthy and costly process and is still a relatively rare occurrence, although the NHS annual compensation bill runs at approximately £500m (NHS Litigation Authority, 2007).

The great majority of patients will usually complain to the nurse's employer or the Nursing & Midwifery Council rather than go to law. However, when a case is successfully brought, an award of significant damages can be made in favour of the patient.

Society

We are all accountable to society through the criminal law. A nurse who breaks the law is as liable to prosecution as any other person. The statutes concerned with the regulation of medicines, such as the Medicines Act 1968 and the Misuse of Drugs Act 1971, carry criminal penalties if breached. It is therefore vital that nurses are within the law when working with medicines.

The four spheres of accountability regulating the practice of the nurse are not mutually exclusive. It is entirely possible that a nurse might be removed from the professional register, be dismissed from post, be sued by a patient and receive a fine, community penalty or imprisonment. It is essential, therefore, that the nurse understands that the notion of accountability is always considered as a whole through all four spheres. This will ensure safe and effective practice, which will benefit the patient and avoid being called to justify one's actions.

REGULATION OF CLINICAL TRIALS

Nurses and their patients need to be confident of the quality and safety of medicines used in practice. In the UK, all medicinal products must be granted a marketing authorisation before they can be sold or prescribed to patients. This authorisation is only granted when the Medicines and Healthcare products Regulatory Agency (MHRA) is satisfied that the drug is safe and effective. Clinical trials are undertaken to allow data on safety and therapeutic effects to be collected and analysed. The trials are conducted with healthy volunteers or patients, depending on the type of medicine and the stage of its development.

The danger to human subjects involved in clinical trials was highlighted by an incident at a trial at Northwick Park Hospital in Hertfordshire in March 2006. Six of the eight participants experienced a life-threatening reaction to the drug being trialled and had to spend several days in intensive care.

To minimise the danger to volunteers, and potentially to the public, from the adverse effects of new untried medicinal compounds, a strict European-wide regulatory framework controls both pre-trial laboratory testing and clinical trial testing on humans to ensure that they are properly designed (Council Directive (EC) 2001/20, 2001).

Since May 2004 all clinical trials are required to meet the standards set by the European Union Clinical Trials Directive (Council Directive (EC) 2001/20, 2001). The directive seeks to harmonise the laws, regulations and administrative provisions of member states in relation to good clinical practice when conducting clinical trials on medicinal products for human use.

In the UK, the Clinical Trials Directive was implemented by the Medicines for Human Use (Clinical Trials) Regulations 2004. The 2004 regulations define a clinical trial as:

Any investigation in human subjects, intended to discover or verify the clinical, pharmacological and or other pharmacodynamic effects of one or more investigational medicinal products and or to identify any adverse reactions to one or more investigational medical product and or to study absorption, distribution, metabolism and excretion of one or more investigational medicinal product(s) with the object of ascertaining its/their safety or effectiveness.

(Medicines for Human Use (Clinical Trials)
Regulations 2004, regulation 2)

From compound to clinical trial

It can take upwards of 15 years to develop and market a new medicinal product. In the early stages pharmaceutical companies are not always certain that a new compound will be effective as a medicine, and during the development process the efficacy of a drug can change to a different therapeutic area. For example, Viagra began as a treatment for angina and its benefit in relation to erectile dysfunction only became apparent after early clinical trials.

Prior to testing in human subjects, unpromising compounds are sifted out and candidate compounds selected for development as investigational medicinal products (IMPs). Non- and pre-clinical laboratory and animal tests are then carried out and analysed before the IMPs are tested in humans using a clinical trial.

A clinical trial of an IMP must have a favourable opinion from an ethics committee and authorisation from the MHRA before it can begin (Medicines for Human Use (Clinical Trials) Regulations 2004, schedule 2). The MHRA is the UK's licensing authority for medicines.

Once approved, the trial will go through four different phases. These are carried out under the strict supervision of doctors, nurses and other health professionals, and enforced by inspections from the MHRA [Medicines for Human Use (Clinical Trials) Regulations 2004, regulation 47].

Phases of a clinical trial

- Phase 1, or healthy volunteers' trials, are small studies and the first test of a drug in humans. They are designed to establish safe or tolerable levels of the drug and the route by which it should be taken. The volunteers must be healthy and usually under the age of 45 years. The trial of the monoclonal antibody TGN1412 at Northwick Park Hospital, which resulted in six volunteers needing intensive care, was a phase 1 trial.
- Phase 2 trials involve groups of 100–200 patients suffering from the disease that the drug is being developed to treat. They provide more evidence about activity and safety, and are also used to define the dosage and regimen for the medicine.
- Phase 3 trials are larger-scale controlled trials designed to assess the risks and benefits of the treatment. Such trials involve 1000–3000 patients, sometimes many more, and compare the treatment under assessment with either a placebo or a comparator drug. It is more usual in UK trials for a comparator drug to be used rather than a placebo as ethics committees tend to consider this a more ethical approach [Association of the British Pharmaceutical Industry (ABPI), 2003].
- Phase 4 trials are those initiated after marketing authorisation has been granted and the medicine has been launched. It allows the effectiveness of the medicine to be assessed in a broad range of patients. Safety is a major part of the phase 4 trial, and the large subject size allows for rarer adverse reactions to be recorded and monitored. Doctors and non-medical prescribers such as district nurses are also able to assess quality-of-life issues and secondary benefits of the medicines. Phase 4 trials also provide an opportunity to develop new uses for the medicine and allow the new product to be compared with other treatments for the condition.

Trial results will be published in academic journals for the benefit of other health professionals interested in the findings and potential new treatments. Where the trial is unfavourable it can prove difficult to have the research accepted for publication; in this case the pharmaceutical industry generally makes alternative publication arrangements through journal supplements, clinical reports, conference papers and the internet so that the data are available for scrutiny to the health and scientific community (ABPI, 2003).

Participation in clinical trials

The type of participant required by researchers for clinical trials depends on the stage of the trial and the nature of the IMP.

Volunteers for phase 1 trials are generally recruited through advertising and, while they can be reimbursed for their expenses, money cannot be used to induce a person to participate (ABPI, 2003).

Patients taking part in phases 2 and 3 of the clinical trial are recruited in a number of ways. Local adverts may be placed in newspapers and on radio, or placed on hospital and GP surgery notice boards. Patients may learn about a clinical trial into their condition through a support group and volunteer to take part. The most likely method of recruitment, however, is through invitation. Doctors and other health professionals, such as district nurses, who are involved with or are aware of a trial of relevance to their patient will invite the patient to participate if they feel it would be in the interest of the patient to do so.

Before participants are enrolled on a trial, they are physically examined by the research team and they continue to be monitored throughout the trial. Whether volunteers are healthy phase 1 participants or persons suffering from the illness the IMP is intended to treat in phases 2 and 3 of the trial, all participants must give their informed consent for entering the trial and are free to withdraw at any time without prejudice to their continuing care (Medicines for Human Use (Clinical Trials) Regulations 2004, schedule 1 part 3).

Consent to participate in clinical trials

Participants in clinical trials generally have to be capable adults who give their informed consent to taking part.

For the purpose of clinical trials, a person gives informed consent to take part only if:

- their decision is given freely;
- they are informed of the nature, significance, implications and risks of the trial;
- the consent is given in writing and dated and signed; or
- if they are unable to sign or mark documents to indicate their consent, they give consent orally in the presence of at least one witness who records it in writing.

(Medicines for Human Use (Clinical Trials) Regulations 2004, schedule 1 part 1 paragraph 3)

Clinical trials and the incapacitated adult

The Medicines for Human Use (Clinical Trials) Regulations 2004 allows for trial participants to be chosen from persons considered to be incapable adults subjected to safeguards.

Research can only be carried out on an adult subject who lacks capacity if:

- there are grounds for expecting that the IMP to be tested will produce a benefit to the subject that outweighs the risks;
- the clinical trial relates directly to a life-threatening or debilitating clinical condition from which the subject suffers;
- the clinical trial is essential to validate data obtained in other clinical trials involving persons able to give consent or the data have been obtained by other research methods.

Where a person lacks the requisite capacity to make a decision, special rules apply concerning permission for that person to participate in a clinical trial. The Medicines for Human Use (Clinical Trials) Regulations 2004 requires the permission of a third party known as a 'legal representative' before the incapable adult can participate in the trial.

Clinical trials and minors

The Medicines for Human Use (Clinical Trials) Regulations 2004 also includes safeguards where children are to be the subjects of a clinical trial. As with incapable adults, a clinical trial with children as subjects will only be sanctioned where:

- it relates directly to a clinical condition from which the minor suffers or it can only be carried out on minors;

- some direct benefit for the group of patients involved in the clinical trial is to be obtained from that trial;
- it is necessary to validate data obtained in other clinical trials involving persons able to give informed consent, or other research methods.

The Medicines for Human Use (Clinical Trials) Regulations 2004 defines a minor as a person under 16 years of age. Before a minor child can participate in a clinical trial, the informed consent of a person representing the child, such as a parent or some other person with parental responsibility, needs to be given.

THE LEGAL REGULATION OF MEDICINES

Medicines Act 1968
The principal statute regulating the use of medicines is the Medicines Act 1968. This provides an administrative and licensing system to control the sale and supply of medicines to the public. Before a drug can be marketed for sale to the public it must have a marketing authorisation issued by the Secretary of State for Health. A marketing authorisation cannot be issued unless the Commission on Human Medicines, under the auspices of the MHRA, has been consulted (section 2, Medicines Act 1968). The MHRA is further charged with the promotion of the collection of data on adverse reactions to drugs (section 4, Medicines Act 1968).

Drugs that have a manufacturing authorisation are categorised into three types for the purpose of supply to the general public:

- *General sales list drugs*: This type of drug may be sold through a variety of outlets without the need for a registered pharmacist. Examples include paracetamol and aspirin.
- *Pharmacy only*: This category of medicine can only be purchased under the supervision of a registered pharmacist in a retail pharmacy. Examples include ranitidine, cimetidine and piriton.
- *Prescription only*: This category of medicine can only be obtained from a registered pharmacist by prescription from a registered doctor, dentist or eligible non-medical prescriber. These drugs cannot normally be supplied unless a prescription

has been issued from an appropriate practitioner. The criteria for determining which products should be available on prescription only are regulated by European Directive 92/26/EEC. These medicines are listed in article 3 of the Prescription Only Medicines (Human Use) Order 1997. Under the Medicines (Products Other Than Veterinary Drugs) (Prescription Only) Order 1983, in exceptional circumstances, pharmacists may supply five days' emergency treatment of a prescription-only product.

Appropriate practitioners

The Medicines Act 1968, section 58(1), bestows prescribing authority to registered medical practitioners, dentists and vets who are able to issue prescriptions from their relevant formularies. The Medicinal Products: Prescribing by Nurses etc. Act 1992 and Health & Social Care Act 2001, section 63, extended the range of appropriate practitioners. The Medicines for Human Use (Prescribing) (Miscellaneous Amendments) Order 2006 introduced three categories of non-medical prescribers:

- independent;
- independent/supplementary;
- community practitioner.

Under the 2006 regulations, registered nurses whose names in each case are held on the Nursing and Nursery Council professional register, with an annotation signifying that they have successfully completed an approved programme of preparation and training, can become independent and/or supplementary prescribers.

Definitions
Administration

This is not generally defined but accepted as involving the drug being given by a practitioner or a practitioner supervising the patient taking the dose. The Prescription Only Medicines (Human Use) Order 1997 defines parenteral administration as administration by breach of the skin or mucous membrane.

Supply
Section 131 of the Medicines Act 1968 defines supply as supplying a drug in circumstances corresponding to retail sale. However, if a nurse were providing any prescription-only medicine for patients to take away and administer themselves, then that would amount to supply. For example, a nurse supplying a medicine under a patient group direction must issue the medicine in a pre-packed form suitable for the patient to take away. The nurse cannot issue a note for a pharmacist to supply the medicine.

Prescription
This means a prescription issued by an appropriate practitioner under or by virtue of the NHS Act 1977. That is, it is written on the proscribed form and is signed and dated by the practitioner, for example FP10.

The form of a prescription
Article 15 of the Prescription Only Medicines (Human Use) Order 1997 requires that a prescription must be completed and signed in ink, or be otherwise indelible, on the statutory form and must contain the following information:

- the name and address of the patient;
- the drug described clearly;
- the signature of the prescriber;
- the date of signing;
- the address of the appropriate practitioner;
- the status of the appropriate practitioner (e.g. nurse independent prescriber).

Administration of prescription-only medicines
A drug categorised as a prescription-only medicine can normally only be administered by or under the direction of an appropriate practitioner. Section 58(2)(b) of the Medicines Act 1968 states that:

No person shall administer otherwise than to himself any such medicinal product unless he is an appropriate practitioner or a person acting in accordance with the directions of an appropriate practitioner.

However, article 9 of the Prescription Only Medicines (Human Use) Order 1997 limits the restriction on the administration of prescription-only medicines to those that are for parenteral administration.

The restriction imposed by s 58(2) (b) shall not apply to the administration to human beings of a prescription only medicine which is not for parenteral administration.

Nurse as appropriate practitioner

The National Health Service (Miscellaneous Amendments Relating to Independent Prescribing) Regulations 2006 introduced independent prescribing and extended the range of medicines that can be prescribed. It allows nurses with this status to prescribe any licensed medicine, including issuing private prescriptions, for any medical condition that an independent prescriber is competent to treat, and this includes some controlled drugs. As appropriate practitioners for the purposes of the Medicines Act 1968, section 58(2), nurses who are independent prescribers can also give directions for the administration of any product they are legally allowed to prescribe, as long as they are satisfied that the person to whom they give the instructions is competent to administer the medicine.

All registered nurses can train to be independent prescribers. However, the NMC Standards of Proficiency (NMC, 2006) for nurse prescribers state that practitioners must have at least 3 years' post-registration experience before undertaking the course. Nurses who successfully complete the programme must register their prescribing qualification with the NMC before they can start prescribing.

Prescribing borderline substances, off-label medicines or unlicensed medicines

Borderline substances are mainly foodstuffs, such as enteral feeds and foods that are specially formulated for people with medical conditions. They also include some toiletries, such as sun blocks. Independent prescribers are able to prescribe these products but should limit their prescriptions to the substances on the Advisory Committee on Borderline Substances approved list, which is published as Part XV of the Drug Tariff and can also be found in the *British National Formulary*.

The terms 'off-label' or 'off-licence' medicines describe the use of licensed medicines in a dose, age group or by a route not in the product specification. Nurses who are independent prescribers can prescribe off label but in doing so take full responsibility for their prescribing. They will be accountable for harm caused to the patient by off-licence prescribing or administration. For example, the Department of Health [Department of Health (DH), 2003] reported an incident of off-license administration where a nurse crushed an antibiotic tablet and inserted it into an intravenous infusion because the patient had swallowing difficulties. The patient collapsed and required four days of therapy in intensive care.

Regardless of the nurse's prescribing authority, an off-licence prescription or administration will not give the practitioner the protection from liability for unsafe products normally given by the Consumer Protection Act 1987 that holds the producer liable for a defective product. Where a patient is harmed by a medicine prescribed or administered off licence then liability in negligence could arise for the practitioner.

Unlicensed medicines are those that do not have a product licence because, for example, there may not be enough commercial interest in marketing the medicine in the UK. This can happen if there are only a very small number of patients who would use the medicine. Such medicines are often available from specialist manufacturers or made up by pharmacists as patient-specific formulations, often known as specials. Independent prescribers cannot prescribe unlicensed medicines.

Supplementary prescribers

Supplementary prescribing was introduced in April 2003 and is a voluntary prescribing partnership between the independent prescriber, who must be a doctor or dentist, and the supplementary prescriber, who can be a nurse, to implement an agreed patient-specific clinical management plan.

The Prescription Only Medicines (Human Use) Order 1997 requires that, to be lawful, supplementary prescribing by a registered nurse must only occur where:

- the independent prescriber is a doctor (or dentist);
- the supplementary prescriber is a registered nurse whose name is recorded in the relevant register with an annotation signifying that they are qualified to order drugs, medicines and appliances as a supplementary prescriber;
- there is a written clinical management plan relating to a named patient and to that patient's specific conditions;
- agreement to the plan is recorded by both the independent prescriber and the supplementary prescriber before it begins;
- the independent prescriber and the supplementary prescriber share access to, consult and use the same common patient record.

Following diagnosis by the doctor and agreement of the clinical management plan, the supplementary prescriber may prescribe any medicine for the patient that is referred to in the plan until the next review by the independent prescriber. There is no formulary for supplementary prescribing and no restrictions on the medical conditions that can be managed under these arrangements. The scope of supplementary prescribing is very broad, and any prescription-only medicine, pharmacy medicine, general sales list medicine or controlled drug, whether licensed or unlicensed, can be issued as long as it is part of the agreed clinical management plan.

The NMC (2006) argues that because of the bureaucracy of developing individual plans for each patient, supplementary prescribing has been used as a blanket authority to prescribe medication. However, the MHRA, which is responsible for ensuring that medicines' law is complied with, states that using the same clinical management plan for all patients with the same condition is unlawful and does not meet the legislative requirements of supplementary prescribing (MHRA, 2003).

To be lawful a clinical management plan must contain:

- the name of the patient to whom the plan relates;
- the illnesses or conditions that may be treated by the supplementary prescriber;
- the date on which the plan is to take effect and when it is to be reviewed by the doctor or dentist who is a party to the plan;

- reference to the class or description of medicinal product that may be prescribed or administered under the plan;
- any restrictions or limitations as to the strength or dose of any product that may be prescribed or administered under the plan, and any period of administration or use of any medicinal product that may be prescribed or administered under the plan;
- relevant warnings about the known sensitivities of the patient to, or known difficulties of the patient with, particular medicinal products;
- the arrangements for notification of:
  - suspected or known adverse reactions to any medicinal product that may be prescribed or administered under the plan;
  - suspected or known adverse reactions to any other medicinal product taken at the same time as any medicinal product prescribed or administered under the plan;
  - the circumstances in which the supplementary prescriber should refer to, or seek the advice of, the doctor or dentist who is a party to the plan.

(Prescription Only Medicines (Human Use) Order 1997)

A supplementary prescriber who issues a prescription in contravention of the regulations could face prosecution under the regulations and a misconduct charge from the NMC as well as disciplinary proceeds from their employer.

The training for supplementary prescribing is incorporated into non-medical independent prescribing courses (NMC, 2006).

Alternatives to prescriptions for the supply and administration of medicines

As well as granting prescribing authority, the Medicines Act 1968 and its regulations allow for the supply and administration of prescription-only medicines by nurses without a prescription through the use of patient-specific directions, patient group directions and specific exemptions under the Prescription Only Medicines (Human Use) Order 1997.

Patient group directions

A patient group direction is a written instruction for the supply or administration of a licensed medicine in an identified clinical situation where the patient may not be individually identified before presenting for treatment. Since 2003, independent hospital agencies and clinics registered under the Care Standards Act 2000, prison healthcare services, police services and defence medical services have also been able to use patient group directions.

A patient group direction is drawn up locally by doctors, pharmacists and other health professionals and must meet the legal criteria set out in Box 2.1.

Box 2.1 Legal requirements for a valid patient group direction

The name of the body to which the direction applies.

The date the direction comes into force and the date it expires.

A description of the medicine(s) to which the direction applies.

The clinical conditions covered by the direction.

A description of those patients excluded from treatment under the direction.

A description of the circumstances under which further advice should be sought from a doctor (or dentist, as appropriate) and arrangements for referral made.

Appropriate dosage and maximum total dosage, quantity, pharmaceutical form and strength, route and frequency of administration, and minimum or maximum period over which the medicine should be administered.

Relevant warnings, including potential adverse reactions.

Details of any follow-up action and the circumstances.

A statement of the records to be kept for audit purposes.

Names and signatures of registered practitioners entitled to supply and/or administer medicines under the patient group direction.

Source: Prescription Only Medicines (Human Use) Amendment Order 2000.

Each patient group direction must be signed by a doctor and a pharmacist, and approved by the organisation in which it is to be used, typically a Primary Care or NHS Trust. Patient group directions can only be used by registered healthcare professionals, including nurses, acting as named individuals, and a list of individuals named as competent to supply and administer medicines under the direction must be included.

A patient group direction can include a flexible dose range for the nurse to select the appropriate dose for the patient. Medicines can also be used off licence provided such use is supported by best clinical practice and the patient group direction contains a statement why this is necessary.

The Misuse of Drugs Regulations 2001 was amended in 2003 to allow some controlled drugs to be supplied and or administered under a patient group direction. These include:

- diamorphine, but only for treatment of cardiac pain by nurses working in coronary care units and accident and emergency departments of hospitals;
- all drugs listed in schedule 4 of the 2001 Regulations (mostly benzodiazepines), except anabolic steroids;
- all drugs listed in schedule 5 of the 2001 Regulations (i.e. low-strength opiates such as codeine).

The National Prescribing Centre (2004) suggests that the supply and administration of medicines under patient group directions should be reserved for the limited number of situations where this offers an advantage for patient care without compromising patient safety. It further suggests that particular caution should be used when deciding whether to use a patient group direction for an antibiotic as antimicrobial resistance is a public health issue of great concern and care should be taken to ensure that any strategy to control increasing resistance will not be jeopardised. For example, a patient group direction should not allow the supply or administration of a medicine for minor viral diseases that are unaffected by antibiotics such as treating sore throats in the absence of good evidence of bacterial infection.

Patient-specific direction

A patient-specific direction is a written instruction for medicines to be supplied for administering to a named patient. Examples are an instruction on a ward drug chart or an instruction by a GP in medical notes for a nurse to administer a medicine.

A patient-specific direction is individually tailored to the needs of a single patient, and it should be used in preference to a patient group direction wherever appropriate.

Authority for patient-specific directions

The Prescription Only Medicines (Human Use) Order 1997 authorises the use of patient-specific directions, and article 12 of the order allows any appropriate practitioner (including nurses with independent prescribing authority) to write a written instruction for the supply and administration of a prescription-only medicine in a hospital.

Article 12A of the 1997 Order gives an exemption for the supply and administration of prescription-only medicines by an NHS body where the medicine is supplied for the purpose of being administered to a particular person in accordance with the written directions of a doctor, even though the direction does not satisfy the conditions for a valid prescription.

A patient-specific direction differs from a prescription. To be lawful, a prescription must meet the requirements of article 15 of the 1997 order. A patient-specific direction is lawful even if it does not meet these requirements, and a nurse is entitled to administer medicines in accordance with a patient-specific direction.

Specific exemption for the supply or administration of medicines under the Medicines Act 1968

The Medicines Act, section 58(2)(b), requires that the administration of a prescription-only medicine be done by or under the direction of an appropriate practitioner. This normally requires a prescription.

Exemption for the administration of a prescription-only medicine in an emergency

A general exemption on restriction from parenteral administration is allowed for medicinal products for the purpose of saving life in an emergency, and there is no specific restriction on who is entitled to administer these medicines. The drugs include adrenaline injection 1 in 1000 (1 mg in 1 ml) and atropine sulphate injection.

Similar arrangements exist for the supply of prescription-only medicines in an emergency.

CONTROLLED DRUGS

Nurses will be familiar with controlled drugs and their valuable contribution to the care of patients, particularly those in severe cardiac pain and those with otherwise intractable pain who are receiving palliative care. However, nurses will also be aware that controlled drugs have the potential to be misused, even by health professionals. The case of Harold Shipman, a doctor convicted of about 15 murders, who is believed to have killed in the region of 260 of his patients over a 30-year period, mainly through the use of lethal injections of controlled drugs, before being detected, highlights the need to ensure that procedures are in place to monitor the storage, recording and use of controlled drugs by health professionals, including nurse prescribers (*R* v *Shipman* [2000]; The Shipman Inquiry, 2004a).

An expansion of non-medical prescribing and amendments to the Misuse of Drugs Regulations 2001 now allow more nurses to prescribe a greater number of controlled drugs to their patients. It is essential, therefore, that nurses are aware of the legal restrictions designed to prevent misuse of controlled drugs, including those introduced following the recommendations of the Shipman Inquiry (2004b), to ensure safer management of controlled drugs.

Parliament recognised, by the early 1970s, the need for comprehensive legislation to control the misuse of drugs and enacted the Misuse of Drugs Act 1971 to make a list of all dangerous or otherwise harmful drugs that were to be subjected to control, and therefore called controlled drugs, and to create a framework to prevent their misuse.

Misuse of Drugs Act 1971

Controlled drugs are listed under schedule 2 of the Misuse of Drugs Act 1971 under one of three classifications:

- *Class A*: These include cocaine and crack cocaine, ecstasy, heroin, LSD, methadone, processed magic mushrooms and any Class B drug that is injected.
- *Class B*: These include amphetamine, barbiturates and codeine.
- *Class C*: These include mild amphetamines, anabolic steroids, and minor tranquillisers and cannabis (in resin, oil or herbal form).

Class A drugs are treated by the law as the most dangerous, and offences involving this class of drug carry the highest penalties.

Restrictions on prescribing and administering controlled drugs

Under the provisions of the Misuse of Drugs Act 1971, it is an offence to supply or possess drugs that are controlled under schedule 2 of that Act. Health professionals would commit these offences unless the law provided for an exemption allowing certain controlled drugs to be used for medicinal and scientific purposes.

The Misuse of Drugs Regulations 2001 in conjunction with the Medicines Act 1968 set out the requirements for the use, possession, storage and recording of controlled drugs for medicinal or scientific use. These regulations allow health professionals to possess and supply a controlled drug whilst performing their duties without committing an offence.

The 2001 Regulations divide controlled drugs into five schedules. Each of the schedules has different licensing and other restrictions regarding the production, distribution and possession of drugs contained within that schedule. The degree of control ranges from virtual absolute prohibition under schedule 1 to almost complete exemption in schedule 5.

Schedule 1 (controlled drugs licence)

Drugs in schedule 1 are the most stringently controlled. Schedule 1 drugs are not authorised for medical use and can only be supplied, possessed or administered by a person authorised by a licence issued by the Home Office. Such licences are granted for research or special purposes. These drugs cannot be prescribed by doctors or dispensed by pharmacists for medicinal use. Drugs in schedule 1 include LSD, cannabis and raw opium.

Schedule 2 (controlled drugs)

Controlled drugs (CD) include the opiates, secobarbital, amphetamine and cocaine, and are subjected to safe custody requirements and so must be stored in a locked receptacle, usually in an appropriate controlled drug cabinet or approved safe, which can only be opened by the person in lawful possession of the controlled drug or a person authorised by that person. The drug may be administered to a patient by a doctor or dentist, or by any person acting in accordance with the directions of a doctor or dentist. A register must be kept for schedule 2 controlled drugs, and this register must comply with the relevant regulations. The destruction of controlled drugs in schedule 2 must be appropriately authorised, and the person witnessing the destruction must be authorised to do so.

Schedule 3 (CD no register)

Medicines in this schedule include a number of minor stimulant drugs and other drugs that are less likely to be misused than the drugs in schedule 2. They are exempt from safe custody requirements and can be stored on the open dispensary shelf except for flunitrazepam, temazepam, buprenorphine and diethylpropion, which must be stored in a locked controlled drug receptacle.

Schedule 3 drugs are subjected to the same special prescribing requirements as those in schedule 2. There is no legal requirement to record schedule 3 transactions in a controlled drug register. In addition, the requirements relating to destruction do not apply unless the controlled drugs are manufactured by the individual. Invoices for these drugs must be retained for a minimum of 2 years.

Schedule 4 (CD benzodiazepines and CD anabolic steroids)

Medicines in this schedule are exempt from safe custody requirements, with destruction requirements only applying to importers, exporters and manufacturers. Specific controlled drug prescription writing requirements do not apply, and controlled drug registers do not need to be kept, although records should be kept if such controlled drugs are produced or if a licensed person imports or exports such drugs.

Part 1 of this schedule concerns controlled drug benzodiazepines that include most of the benzodiazepines, plus eight other substances, including fencamfamin and mesocarb. Possession of these drugs is an offence without an appropriate prescription. Possession by practitioners and pharmacists acting in their professional capacities is authorised.

Part 2 concerns controlled drug anabolic steroids and includes most of the anabolic and androgenic steroids, such as testosterone, together with clenbuterol and growth hormones.

There is no restriction on possession when it is part of a medicinal product. A Home Office licence is required for the importation and exportation of these drugs unless the substance is in the form of a medicinal product and is for self-administration by a person.

Schedule 5 (CD invoice)

This schedule includes preparations of certain controlled drugs, for example codeine, pholcodine and morphine, which are exempt from full control when present in medicinal products of low strengths as their risk of misuse is reduced. These non-injectable, small-dose preparations can be purchased over the counter at a pharmacy without prescription, but once obtained it is unlawful for them to be supplied to another person. Many of these preparations include well-known cough mixtures and pain killers. There is no restriction on the import, export, possession, administration or destruction of these preparations, and safe custody regulations do not apply.

A practitioner, pharmacist or person holding an appropriate licence may manufacture or compound any controlled drug in schedule 5. Invoices for these preparations must be kept for a minimum of 2 years.

Nurses and controlled drugs

Nurses, including those with prescribing authority, may lawfully supply controlled drugs to patients in a number of different ways.

Following the introduction of the Misuse of Drugs (Amendment) Regulations 2005, independent nurse prescribers are able to prescribe a range of controlled drugs under specific conditions, as outlined above.

The Misuse of Drugs (Amendment) Regulations 2005 also added supplementary prescribers to the list of people authorised to write prescriptions for controlled drugs, providing they are acting in accordance with a clinical management plan. A further amendment to the General Medical & Pharmaceutical Services Regulations (National Health Service (General Medical Services Contracts) (Personal Medical Services Agreements) and (Pharmaceutical Services) (Amendment) Regulations, 2005) allowed supplementary prescribers to begin to prescribe controlled drugs.

There are no other restrictions on which controlled drugs from schedules 2 to 5 of the 2001 Regulations supplementary prescribers are entitled to prescribe, and it can be seen that, subject to the clinical management plan, supplementary nurse prescribers are entitled to prescribe a wider range of controlled drugs that the limited list available to independent nurse prescribers. Certain nurses may also supply and administer controlled drugs in accordance with a patient group direction.

Safer management of controlled drugs

The devastating consequences of the misuse of controlled drugs by health professionals has been highlighted by the Shipman Inquiry (2004b), which found that inappropriate practice could take several forms:

- dishonest prescribing;
- supplying controlled drugs for monetary gain;
- obtaining controlled drugs to feed the doctor's addiction;
- irresponsible prescribing;
- unwise prescribing;
- self-prescribing or prescribing for family and friends;
- prescribing for 'casual' or occasional patients.

The inquiry therefore made a number of recommendations to strengthen the prescribing of controlled drugs and to monitor their movement from prescriber to dispenser to patient.

Amendments to the Misuse of Drugs Regulations 2001 now allow all details of prescriptions for controlled drugs except the signature to be computer generated, but such prescriptions must show CD after the order for a controlled drug; e.g. diamorphine 10 mg tablets CD (see Box 2.2).

Registers for drugs listed in schedules 1 and 2 of the 2001 Regulations can also be computerised (see Box 2.3).

Further changes came into force in 2006 that focus on strengthening safeguards to prevent misuse of controlled drugs by health professionals. These require that arrangements for dispensing of NHS prescriptions for schedule 2 and 3 controlled drugs by community pharmacists need patients or other people collecting medicines on their behalf to sign for them. The validity of any

---

Box 2.2 A prescription for schedule 2 and 3 CDs

A prescription for schedule 2 and 3 CDs (with the exception of temazepam and preparations containing it) must:

- contain the following details, written so as to be indelible (e.g. written by hand, typed or computer-generated):
  - The patient's full name, address and, where appropriate, age.
  - The name and form of the drug, even if only one form exists.
  - The strength of the preparation, where appropriate.
  - The dose to be taken.
  - The total quantity of the preparation, or the number of dose units, to be supplied in both words and figures.
- be signed by the prescriber with their usual signature (this must be handwritten) and dated by them (the date does not have to be handwritten);
- state that the drug is for dental treatment only if the prescriber is a dentist.

It is also a legal requirement under the Medicines Act 1968 that all prescriptions for prescription-only medicines contain particulars that indicate whether the appropriate practitioner is a doctor, dentist, supplementary prescriber or independent nurse prescriber.

Box 2.3 Recording requirements for controlled drugs

Records for schedule 2 CDs must be kept in a CD register. This is not a legal requirement for schedule 3, 4 or 5 CDs The register must:

- be bound (not loose-leaved) or a computerised system that is in accordance with the best practice guidance endorsed by the Secretary of State under section 2 of the NHS Act 1977;
- contain individual sections for each individual drug;
- have the name of the drug specified at the top of each page;
- have the entries in chronological order and made on the day of the transaction or the next day;
- have the entries made in ink or otherwise so as to be indelible or in a computerised form in which every such entry is attributable and capable of being audited and is in accordance with best practice guidance endorsed by the Secretary of State under section 2 of the NHS Act 1977;
- not have cancellations, obliterations or alterations; corrections must be made by a signed and dated entry in the margin or at the bottom of the page;
- be kept at the premises to which it relates and be available for inspection at any time.

A separate register must:

- be kept for each set of premises;
- be kept for a minimum of 2 years after the date of the last entry, once completed;
- not be used for any other purpose.

For CDs received into stock the following details must be recorded in the CD register:

- the date on which the CD was received;
- the name and address of the supplier (e.g. wholesaler, pharmacy);
- the quantity received;
- the name, form and strength of the CD.

Continued

For CDs supplied to patients (via prescriptions) or to practitioners (via requisitions), the following details must be recorded in the CD register:

- the date on which the supply was made;
- the name and address of the patient or practitioner receiving the CD;
- particulars of the authority of person who prescribed or ordered the CD;
- the quantity supplied;
- the name, form and strength in which the CD was supplied.

prescription for schedule 2, 3 and 4 controlled drugs is restricted to 28 days, and the maximum quantity on prescription is limited to 30 days.

All healthcare providers holding stocks of controlled drugs must have and comply with the terms of an agreed standard operating procedure (SOP) that will include regular (monthly) audits of controlled drug stocks and a thorough investigation of any discrepancies.

Palliative care

The key aims of the Shipman Inquiry recommendations are to prevent misuse of controlled drugs by inappropriate prescribing practice. Nurses must also ensure that their administration of controlled drugs meets legal and professional standards, particularly where large doses of controlled drugs are used to control pain in palliative care. Failing to meet these standards, resulting in harm to or the death of a patient, could render nurse prescribers liable to prosecution. Any care or treatment given to a patient that is motivated by a desire to bring about a patient's death is unlawful (Mental Capacity Act 2005 , section 4). In *R* v *Cox* (1992), a consultant rheumatologist was convicted of attempted murder after he admitted injecting a patient with potassium chloride to end her life of pain and suffering. Similarly, in *R* v *Salisbury* [2005] the Court of Appeal accepted that a ward sister had administered controlled drugs to her patients with the intention of killing them.

The principle of double effect

The courts do recognise that nobody should die in pain and that effective palliative care can require what seems like very high doses of analgesia and sedation in the form of controlled drugs. Under the principle of double effect, the courts accept that high doses of controlled drugs may be used to manage pain even though the dose of the drug is likely to harm or even hasten the death of the patient (*Airedale NHS Trust* v *Bland* [1993]; *Pretty* v *DPP* [2001]).

In *R* v *Moor* [2000] the Court accepted that a doctor had used high doses of controlled drugs to relieve pain under the principle of double effect and that he was not motivated by a desire to kill patients. More recently, a doctor accused of giving his patients six times the normal dose of controlled drug was also acquitted of murder by a jury who accepted that he was administering the drugs under the principle of double effect (Strokes, 2005).

It is essential, therefore, that nurses do not prescribe or administer controlled drugs to patients through a desire to bring about those patients' death. Such action is unlawful and prosecution for murder could result.

CIVIL LIABILITY OF NURSES WHEN MANAGING MEDICINES

Negligence

Considerable flexibility is afforded to nurses in the supply and administration of medicines during the course of their practice. The standard required of the nurse is that of the 'ordinary [person] professing to have and exercise that particular skill or art' (J. McNair in *Bolam* v *Friern HMC* [1957]). The House of Lords in *Whitehouse* v *Jordan* [1981] confirmed that this standard applied to errors in the course of treatment, including medication errors.

Parenteral administration of medicines usually involves the use of an injection. The breaking of a needle during an injection is a matter that would require an explanation but has not to date given rise to liability in negligence, but failure to deal with the aftermath of a broken needle has done so. In *Gerber* v *Pines* (1939), a GP was held to be negligent for failing to inform a woman that a piece of needle remained in her after it broke during an injection. In *Horler* v *Kingston and Esher Health Authority* [1993], a surgeon was found negligent after causing scarring when he persisted in trying to remove a needle that broke during suturing. Negligence can also occur where a practitioner injects into the wrong site.

Failure in communication in relation to drug administration has also been shown to be negligent. In *Collins* v *Hertfordshire County Council* (1947), the mishearing of a prescription resulted in a lethal dose being administered and allowing the administration of four extra injections of streptomycin above the 30 prescribed, resulting in permanent loss of balance, rendered a ward sister liable in negligence (*Smith* v *Brighton & Lewes Hospital Management Committee* (1958)).

In *Dwyer* v *Rodrick* (1983), a doctor was found liable in negligence when an incorrectly written prescription resulted in an overdose of the drug. Similarly in *Prendergast* v *Sam & Dee Ltd* (1989), both the doctor and the pharmacist were found liable in negligence when an illegibly written prescription resulted in the wrong drug being supplied to the patient.

A further failure in communication that can render a nurse liable in negligence is a failure to inform a patient of the side effects of a drug. In *Goorkani* v *Tayside Health Board* (1991), a man who had already lost the sight of one eye was given drug therapy to prevent deterioration in the other eye. His doctor did not warn him that the drug carried the risk of infertility as a side effect of long-term prescription, and he became infertile. The court held that the doctor had failed in his duty of care to warn his patient of the risk of infertility arising from extended treatment. It is hoped that this book will assist the nurses by outlining the common adverse reactions and risks associated with medicines commonly used by nurses.

CONSENT ISSUES

The law also regulates the standard of administration through the law of consent. The right to self-determination allows every human being of adult years and sound mind a right to determine what shall be done with their body, and a person has the legal right to accept or decline medical treatment, including medicines (*Airedale NHS Trust* v *Bland* [1993]).

Even though a medicine has been prescribed, it can only be given to a person with their consent. That person has a right to refuse the medication, and those caring for them must respect that right.

Capacity in law is the ability to understand and make a balanced decision and is the key to autonomy (*Re T (Adult: Refusal of Treatment)* [1992]). If a person has capacity, nurses are bound by their decision; if not, the Mental Capacity Act 2005 can allow another person to make that decision or require the nurse to determine if the care and treatment is in their patients' best interests.

The Mental Capacity Act 2005

The Mental Capacity Act 2005 sets out a framework for acting for and making decisions on behalf of people aged 16 years and above who lack the mental capacity to make decisions for themselves. It provides a mechanism for decision making relating the care and treatment of an incapacitated person.

The guiding principles

To underline the Act's fundamental concepts, section 1 establishes a number of statutory principles that must apply to all actions and decisions taken on behalf of a person with incapacity. Nurses will be required to apply these principles when providing care and treatment for a person who is incapable.

- A person must be assumed to have capacity unless it is established that they lack capacity.

  This principle upholds the autonomy of the person. It also means that as the presumption in law is that a person has capacity you do not need to assess the capacity of each woman you care for. You are only required to assess capacity where there is a doubt in your mind about a woman's ability to make a decision.

- A person is not to be treated as unable to make a decision unless all practicable steps to help them to do so have been taken without success.

The test for capacity requires a person to understand and use the treatment information given to them by the nurse. A nurse could render half their patients incapable by explaining treatment in complex terms. This principle requires you to use simple practical steps to support the person, such as a language the person understands, using pictures rather than words, waiting until the person is more alert, etc.

- A person is not to be treated as unable to make a decision merely because they make an unwise decision.

The test for capacity requires that you are able to discern an impairment or disturbance to the persons' mind or brain that might be affecting their decision making ability. Where there is no impairment then you cannot take action under the Mental Capacity Act and must accept the decision as an unwise decision. Recently a young mother refused, on religious grounds, a blood transfusion shortly after giving birth to twins. There was no impairment to the mind or brain and although we might consider it an unwise decision she was entitled to refuse the blood and sadly died.

- An act done or decision made under the Mental Capacity Act for or on behalf of a person who lacks capacity must be done, or made, in the person's best interests.

The Act makes it possible for many people to make decisions on behalf of incapable adults.

- Before the act is done, or the decision is made, regard must be had to whether the purpose for which it is needed can be as effectively achieved in a way that is less restrictive of the person's rights and freedom of action.

Decision-making capacity

Capacity to make decisions is the key to a person's autonomy, and the Mental Capacity Act 2005 sets out a test for decision-making capacity and the circumstances where a person would be regarded as incapable of making a decision. The Act sets out a two-stage functional test based on the decision to be made at the time rather than a person's theoretical ability to make decisions generally. A nurse will need to determine:

- if there is an impairment of or disturbance in the functioning of the person's mind or brain and if there is,

- how far it is affecting the person's ability to make a decision?

The Act also sets out a test for assessing whether a person is unable to make a decision.

Under the provisions of the Mental Capacity Act 2005, a person is unable to make a decision if they are unable to:

- understand the information relevant to the decision;
- retain that information;
- use or weigh that information as part of the process of making the decision;
- communicate the decision (whether by talking, using sign language or any other means).

Even when person has been assessed as lacking decision-making capacity, treatment cannot proceed unless it is in the person's best interests. The Act makes it clear that, 'an act done, or decision made, under this Act for or on behalf of a person who lacks capacity must be done, or made, in his best interests' (Mental Capacity Act 2005, section 1(5)).

The Mental Capacity Act 2005 now provides a checklist of factors that must be considered when determining whether care and treatment are in the best interests of a patient who lacks capacity. This broader, holistic approach ensures that the wishes of the patient and views of those caring for the patient are taken into account.

The Mental Capacity Act 2005 has two formal powers that might allow a third party to make decisions on behalf of a person who lacks decision-making capacity. These powers can give the designated decision maker the right to consent to or refuse medical treatment. Where designated decision makers with authority are in place, their consent must be obtained before care and treatment can lawfully be given, and it is for them to decide whether the care and treatment proposed is in the patient's best interests.

Personal welfare lasting power of attorney

A power allowing another to consent on behalf of a person who lacks capacity can be created through a personal welfare lasting power of attorney. The power must be created by the person when they are capable and will come into force when the person lacks capacity and the power of attorney has been registered with the office of public guardian.

Court of Protection deputy

When continuing decisions need to be made on behalf of a person who lacks capacity and there is no lasting power of attorney then the Court of Protection may appoint a person, called a deputy, to make personal welfare decisions on behalf of the incapable patient, which can include the right to consent to or refuse treatment.

Both the attorney and the deputy must make their decisions in the best interests of the patient. If a nurse believes that a decision is not in the patient's best interests then they may challenge it and try to resolve it with the decision maker. In serious cases, an unresolved dispute may have to be settled by the Court of Protection (Department for Constitutional Affairs, 2007).

The nurse as decision maker

In the absence of a person with the authority to make decisions under the Act's formal powers, the determination of a patient's best interests will fall to the nurse providing the care and treatment to the person who lacks capacity.

Determining a best interest

The checklist of factors to be considered when determining best interests requires the nurse to:

- consider all the relevant circumstances and whether the decision can wait until the person regains capacity;
- so far as reasonably practicable, permit and encourage the person to participate in their care and treatment;

  It is necessary to keep the patient informed by explaining what is happening using all possible means to encourage the person's involvement and participation and upholding their rights and freedoms.

  Consent is a defence to an allegation of trespass to the person and a pragmatic clinical requirement that acknowledges that care and treatment requires the cooperation of the patient if it is to be carried out successfully, therefore even if the person lacks capacity to make a decision, encouraging cooperation will make delivering care and treatment more efficient and effective (*Re W (A Minor) (Medical Treatment: Court's Jurisdiction)* [1993]).

- not be motivated by a desire to bring about the death of the patient;

    All reasonable steps that are in the persons' best interests should be taken to prolong their life unless treatment is futile, overly burdensome to the patient or there is no prospect of recovery (Department for Constitutional Affairs, 2007).

- consider, so far as is reasonably ascertainable:
  - the person's past and present wishes and feelings (and, in particular, any relevant written statement made when they had capacity);

      Nurses are required to make every attempt to discover the person's current wishes and feelings whether this is expressed in words or in behaviour. For example, the display of considerable distress when treating an incapable adult might lead the nurse to conclude that the care and treatment are not in a person's best interests.
  - the beliefs and values that would be likely to influence their decision if they had capacity;

      Equally important are the person's values and beliefs indicated by their cultural background and known past behaviour or expressions, such as a religious or a political conviction, for example the person is a Jehovah's Witness who has previously refused blood transfusions.
  - other factors that they would be likely to consider if they were able to do so.
- take into account, if it is practicable and appropriate to consult them, the views of:
  - anyone named by the person as someone to be consulted on the matter in question or on matters of that kind;
  - anyone engaged in caring for the person or interested in the person's welfare;
  - any donee of a lasting power of attorney granted by the person;

○ any deputy appointed for the person by the court.

Where practicable and appropriate the Act requires a consultation to take place with anyone named by the person and anyone engaged in caring for the person or interested in that person's welfare. Nurses will need to show that they have thought carefully about whom to consult and be prepared to explain why a consultation that they declined to carry out was either impracticable or inappropriate.

The aim of the checklist is to assist nurses who have to make a decision to decide whether in all the circumstances available to them the proposed care and treatment are in the person's best interests.

Independent mental capacity advocate

Where no suitable person is available to be consulted by the nurse on the best interests of the patient then a duty to instruct an independent mental capacity advocate (IMCA) will arise where the decision concerns serious medical treatment, i.e.involves providing, withdrawing or withholding treatment in the following circumstances:

- In a case where a single treatment is being proposed, there is a fine balance between its benefits to the patient and the burdens and risks it is likely to entail.
- In a case where there is a choice of treatments, a decision as to which one to use is finely balanced.
- What is proposed would be likely to involve serious consequences for the patient.

(The Mental Capacity Act 2005
(Independent Mental Capacity Advocate)
(General) Regulations 2006)

The nurse must instruct and consult an IMCA, who will make representations about the person's wishes, feelings and beliefs and call the decision maker's attention to the factors relevant to their decision. The IMCA has the right to see the patient in private and to have access to relevant health records.

Circumstances where the best interests doctrine does not apply

The best interest doctrine does not apply where patients have set out care and treatment they wish to refuse in a valid and applicable advance decision refusing treatment. The nurse would be obliged to respect the wishes of the patient and withhold the treatment.

Crushing tablets

A decision to crush tablets is generally based on one of the following reasons:

- to disguise the administration of the medicine;
- to assist a patient with swallowing difficulties to take the medication.

Covert administration of medicines

The principle of self-determination requires that respect is given to the wishes of the patient. If a capable adult patient refuses, however, to consent to treatment or care, those responsible for the patient's care must respect the patient's wishes, even if they do not consider it to be in the best interests of the patient to do so (*Airedale NHS Trust* v *Bland* (1993)).

Crushing a tablet to disguise its administration from a capable adult would be a trespass to the person in the same way that non-consensual touching would be unlawful. Where a person is unable to consent due to incapacity, the law allows medication to be given, in their best interests, in the absence of a valid consent.

Here, covert administration by crushing a tablet may occur if shown to be safe and in the person's best interests. If not, then the nurse will be held to account. For example, a nurse was removed from the register when found guilty of forcing a patient to swallow a tablet hidden in a marshmallow (NMC, 2002).

In the case of covert administration to an incapable adult, a nurse would need to demonstrate that:

- the patient is incapable of consenting to the treatment;
- the medication is convincingly shown to be therapeutically necessary in the patient's best interests;

- the decision to administer covertly accords with a practice accepted by a responsible body of professional opinion in that it can be shown that:
  - all other methods of administration have been unsuccessfully tried;
  - the pharmacist and those who have to administer the medication agree on the method to be used;
  - the form of the drug is safe to use covertly.

Medication, especially in tablet form, will usually need to be crushed if it is to be administered covertly and disguised in food or drink. Nurses must ensure that no harm will result from food–drug interactions. For example, ampicillin taken with food is likely to have its therapeutic effect fail as it is destroyed by stomach acid. Mixing frusemide with food can result in altered diuresis as absorption is impaired by food (Jordan *et al.*, 2003).

Best practice advice

The NMC's (2007a) revised position statement on the covert administration of medicines reminds nurses that their code of professional conduct requires them to act at all times in such a manner as to justify public trust and confidence. The NMC points out that by disguising medication in food or drink, nurses are acting contrary to that requirement of the code as the patient is being led to believe that they are not receiving medication, when in fact they are.

Covert administration can therefore only be sanctioned where it is convincingly shown to be in the best interests of an incapable patient. It cannot be sanctioned merely because it is easier for the nurse or care team to administer medication in this way.

The requirements of the NMC's position statement on covert administration of medicines are summarised in Box 2.4.

The NMC also requires that local policies regarding covert administration of medicine be developed in accordance with their position statement and the code of professional conduct (NMC, 2007a).

The patient with swallowing difficulties

Crushing a tablet to assist a person with swallowing difficulties appears at first glance to be a less contentious issue. Difficulty

---

Box 2.4 Guidance on the covert administration of medication

Carefully reflect on the reasons for disguising medication and be satisfied that it is necessary:

- to save life;
- to prevent deterioration;
- to ensure an improvement in the patient's physical or mental health.

Ensure that you have the support of the rest of the multiprofessional team.

Do not make a decision to administer medication covertly in isolation.

Record in the patient's care plan all discussions and resulting action regarding the decision to administer medication covertly.

Summarised from NMC (2007) *Covert Administration of Medicines – Disguising Medicine in Food and Drink*. NMC, London.

---

swallowing tablets is one of the most common problems affecting medication compliance among patients. Nurses will commonly encounter patients with swallowing difficulties that will need to be managed if medication adherence is to be achieved.

A frequent solution to a patient's tablet-swallowing problems is to advise crushing the tablet, but tablet crushing carries significant risks and nurses must carefully weigh these risks with their patients before advising them to crush tablets. The NMC (2007b, 2008c) has issued advice for registered nurses and standards for medicines management on the issue of tablet crushing. The regulatory body reminds nurses that they have a responsibility to deliver safe and effective care based on current evidence, best practice and, where applicable, validated research. It therefore advises nurses not to crush any medication or open capsules that are not specifically designed for that purpose, as by doing so the chemical properties of the medication could be altered.

The crushing of a tablet before administration in most cases renders its use unlicensed. Consequently, the manufacturer may assume no liability for any ensuing harm that may come to the patient or the person administering it (Consumer Protection Act, 1987). Where harm is caused as a result of the tablet being altered by crushing, it will not be the producer who is liable but the person who crushed or advised the crushing of the tablet.

Under the Medicines Act 1968, only medical practitioners can authorise the administration of unlicensed medicines to humans. It is therefore unlawful to crush a tablet before administration without the authorisation of the independent prescriber (NMC, 2007b).

IMPORTANCE OF RECORD KEEPING

A recent report by the National Patient Safety Agency (NPSA) into approximately 60 000 medication incidents in the NHS highlights the importance of keeping accurate records and successfully demonstrating that the duty of care owed by nurses to their patients has been properly discharged (NPSA, 2007).

The key issues of medicine safety to emerge from analysis of medication incidents in the community included communication and documentation, particularly in relation to vaccines, and the transfer of care between the community and hospitals.

With about £500 m in compensation being paid from medication-related errors, the report provides a reminder of the importance of health records as evidence.

Purpose

The main purpose of keeping records is to have an account of the care and treatment given to a patient. This allows progress to be monitored and a clinical history to be developed. The clinical record allows for continuity of care by facilitating treatment and support. It is an integral part of care that is every bit as important as the direct care provided to patients.

As well as their clinical function, records have a very important legal purpose as they provide evidence of your involvement with a patient. They need to be sufficiently detailed to demonstrate this involvement. For example, in *Saunders* v *Leeds Western HA* [1993] a fit four-year-old child suffered cardiac arrest and brain damage during an arthroplasty operation. The theatre team argued that the patient's pulse had simply stopped abruptly. Following expert evidence this was rejected by the court. As there was no evidence in the records of a sequence of events leading to the pulse stopping, the court found the health authority liable in negligence.

In civil cases the standard of proof is the balance of probability, i.e. if the weight of evidence is 51% in your favour the case is won. As a nurse's contact with patients is mainly on a one-to-one basis, records made at the time of or soon after seeing a patient often provide the evidence needed to win the case. For example, in *McLennan* v *Newcastle HA* [1992] a patient claimed she had not been told of the relatively high risk associated with her operation. The surgeon, however, had written in the notes at the time that the risks were explained and understood by the patient. This contemporaneous record persuaded the judge that the patient had probably been told about the risks and the case failed.

What to include

Record keeping must not be viewed as a mechanistic process. What you write does matter. In litigation the outcome is not based on truth but proof. If it is not in the notes it can be difficult to prove that it happened. Cases are won and lost on the strength of records. Records are rarely neutral; they will either support or condemn you. You must approach record keeping with the possibility of the records being used in court as evidence.

Records need to be sufficiently detailed to show that you have discharged your duty of care. An evidence-based care plan and regular progress reports form the backbone of this detail. In *Marriott* v *West Midlands HA* [1999] a GP was found negligent when he failed to refer back to hospital a man who had suffered a head injury in a fall and was still having headaches, lethargy and appetite loss a week later. As this was a home visit, the GP had not taken the man's records and was heavily hampered in court by not being able to recount the detail and results of the examination he carried out or why he had decided not to refer the patient back to hospital.

In *Marriott* v *West Midlands HA* [1999] an incomplete and inaccurate record was fatal to the case. Details of the examination were missing but equally damning was the lack of evidence as to why the doctor decided to wait and see. This type of decision about care must also be included in the patient's record. These decisions are often made on a multidisciplinary basis, and your record should include the background to the discussion with colleagues and the patient and its outcome. This will indicate the reason for the decision and corroborate the account of other team members. Records must also corroborate any other legal requirement or form completed by the patient in your presence. For example, if a patient signs a consent form it should also be recorded and the details discussed included. Details of telephone calls made, even if unanswered, to the patient or to others about the patient and discussions arising from them with date and time should be included, as should referrals to specialist practitioners. When a call is made to another agency on a point of concern, that telephone call should be noted and followed up in writing to provide evidence of the action you have taken.

Similar corroboration should be made where a nurse has made an adverse reaction report under the yellow card scheme. A record entry should be made of the nature of the reaction, the action taken to remedy it and details of the yellow card report submitted (Pirmohamed *et al.*, 2004).

Corroboration of prescribing

The corroboration of a prescription issued by a nurse prescriber is an essential entry in a patient's record. A note of the prescription must be entered into the patient's record as soon as possible after it is issued. The entry must include:

- the name of the prescriber;
- their prescribing status;
- details of the consultation;
- the name of the medicine prescribed;
- the medicine's formulation (tablet, liquid, etc.);
- the medicine's strength;
- the dose;
- the route of administration;
- the quantity prescribed.

Common patient record

Nurses who are supplementary prescribers are required to make entries into a common patient record together with the independent prescriber to improve patient safety. Arrangements for the sharing of the patient record must be put into place at the same time as the supplementary prescribing partnership is set up (DH, 2005). Where they also keep their own nursing record, a similar contemporaneous entry must be made. This will ensure effective communication across the care team.

Legibility

The standard of your handwriting is a part of your duty of care towards a patient. If care is initiated by you through a care plan and harm results because others could not read your writing, then liability in negligence is likely to arise. A good analogy is the case of *Prendergast* v *Sam and Dee* [1989] where an illegible prescription resulted in the patient being given the wrong drug, and this caused harm. The pharmacist was held to be 75% liable for that harm. For the poor handwriting the GP was found to be 25% liable. The Court of Appeal held that there is a duty to write clearly so that busy or careless staff can read your instructions. Legibility extends to the signature of the person who made the entry. Identifying the people and therefore witnesses involved in an incident is crucial to building a successful case.

Writing with indelible ink or typeface is essential for two reasons. Firstly, the record must stand the test of time. It may be many years before it is referred to again, and a faded record is of little value as evidence. In *Reynolds* v *North Tyneside Health Authority* [2002], a case alleging negligence by a midwife at the birth of a child was brought 21 years after the incident. Secondly, the credibility of your record as evidence is enhanced by its being made at the time of the incident. Indelible ink or typeface reassures the court that the entry has not been subsequently altered in any way.

Clarity

Records are an essential tool for the continuity of care. Care to be implemented and progress made must be clearly stated. The record is also likely to be read by patients, as under the Data

Protection Act 1998 patients have the right to access records and obtain an explanation of their contents.

The temptation to use jargon and abbreviations as a form of professional shorthand is compelling for busy health professionals. The risk of miscommunication increases dramatically by using this shorthand. Marsh & Narain (2003) report that a combination of shorthand instructions and poor handwriting lead to the death of a patient. The patient was taking 1 mg of warfarin daily. When reviewed, the GP wrote 'same' on the card. The receptionist mistook the 's' as a '5', and the rest of the word as 'mg', resulting in the patient being given 5 mg of warfarin daily. He died from a massive haemorrhage about 3 weeks later.

Jargon is also used to convey offensive remarks unrelated to patient care. Brindley (2003) reports the use of offensive cryptic acronyms such as FLK for 'funny-looking kid' often explained by JLD or 'just like dad'. In litigation, records will be subjected to rigorous scrutiny. There is no right to withhold any part of the record from the court. Having to explain offensive jargon or acronyms under cross-examination will be at best embarrassing and at worst fatal to the case. Evidentially the first impression the court has of you is from your notes. If records are not professional then the assumption is that the care isn't either, and your credibility as a witness is greatly diminished.

Accuracy

To confirm the chronology of record entries, each entry must be identified with the date (day, month and year) and time (using the 24-hour clock), and signed with the professional's name printed legibly underneath the signature together with their position. All alterations must be made by scoring out with a single line that does not completely obscure the error. Correcting fluid must not be used. This removes any suggestion of wrong doing or attempting to cover up an incident. The struck-out error should be followed by the dated, timed and signed correct entry. No blank lines or spaces that could facilitate entries being added at a later date should be left between entries.

Contemporaneous record keeping

Record entries need to be written at the time of or as soon as possible after the events to which they relate. Contemporaneous recording is vital as it adds to the reliability of the entry and means that with the leave of the court you can refer to the record when giving evidence. Contemporaneous altering of a record contributed to a finding of negligence in *Kent* v *Griffiths & Others* [2000]. Here an emergency ambulance took about 30 minutes to arrive at an address of a woman in labour suffering an asthma attack. The crew recorded the duration of the journey as 9 minutes. The judge held that the record had been contemporaneously falsified and found for the patient.

The DH (2005) recommends that an entry corroborating prescribing activity must be made within 48 hours of the prescription. If it is argued that pressure of work so drained available resources that the standard of care was lowered, the court can look at the records of other patients seen on that day to corroborate this.

In *Deacon* v *McVicar* (1984), the judge ordered disclosure of the notes of other patients in a hospital to see how busy staff were on a particular evening. The records of the other patients confirmed that it was an unusually busy time and the case was decided in the hospital's favour.

Records are rarely neutral. Their importance as evidence is such that they will either support you or condemn you. Incomplete or inaccurate records will diminish your credibility as a witness and make it easier for the court to find against you.

In *S (A Child)* v *Newcastle & North Tyneside HA* [2001], the negligent management of the latter stages of labour resulted in severe cerebral palsy. The judge's annoyance at the standard of record keeping is clear from his comments:

It is important to emphasise at this early stage that unhappily the evidence was, in certain important respects, incomplete. The clinical records of this labour are not full and no records at all appear between 4 a.m. and 10.15 a.m. Each of these might be regarded as critical periods. Unhappily whoever did take over from [the midwife] singularly failed to complete the partogram which is effectively devoid of useful information …

The court found in favour of the child.

Audit

Audit is by far the best method of improving and sustaining a high standard of record keeping. The Audit Commission (2002), in its review of health records, found that subjecting records to audit cuts down dramatically on errors and poor standards.

Nurses must subject their records for audit to ensure that they meet the criteria for reliable evidence and discharge of duty.

CONCLUSION

- The law regulates the arrangements for the supply and administration of medicines to patients.
- To practise safely and avoid legal and professional liability, nurses must ensure that they manage medicines properly and have the proper authority to prescribe or administer.
- All medicinal products must be granted a marketing authorisation before they can be sold or prescribed to patients.
- To minimise the danger to volunteers and, potentially, the public from the adverse effects of new untried medicinal compounds, a strict European-wide regulatory framework controls both pre-trial laboratory testing and clinical trial testing.
- The Medicines Act 1968 provides an administrative and licensing system to control the sale and supply of medicines to the public.
- Borderline substances are mainly foodstuffs, such as enteral feeds and foods that are specially formulated for people with medical conditions.
- The terms 'off-label' or 'off-licence' medicines describe the use of licensed medicines in a dose, in an age group or by a route not in the product specification.
- Unlicensed medicines are those that do not have a product licence because there may not be enough commercial interest in marketing the medicine in the UK.
- A patient group direction is a written instruction for the supply or administration of a licensed medicine in an identified clinical situation where the patient may not be individually identified before presenting for treatment.
- A patient-specific direction is a written instruction for medicines to be supplied for administering to a named patient.

- A general exemption on restriction from administration of prescription-only medicines is allowed for the purpose of saving life in an emergency and there is no specific restriction on who is entitled to administer these medicines.
- The Misuse of Drugs Act 1971 and its regulations list all dangerous or otherwise harmful drugs, called controlled drugs, and creates a framework to prevent their misuse.
- The Misuse of Drugs Regulations 2001 in conjunction with the Medicines Act 1968 set out the requirements for the use, possession, storage and recording of controlled drugs for medicinal or scientific use.
- The standard required of the nurse is that of the ordinary person professing to have and exercise that particular skill or art.
- The law also regulates the standard of administration through the law of consent.
- A decision to crush tablets is generally taken to disguise the administration of the medicine or assist a patient with swallowing difficulties to take the medication.
- Covert administration can only be sanctioned where it is convincingly shown to be in the best interests of an incapable patient.
- Nurses must not crush any medication or open capsules that are not specifically designed for that purpose, as by doing so the chemical properties of the medication could be altered.
- The main purpose of keeping records is to have an account of the care and treatment given to a patient.
- Audit is by far the best method of improving and sustaining a high standard of record keeping.

REFERENCES

Airedale NHS Trust v *Bland* [1993] AC 789.

Association of the British Pharmaceutical Industry (ABPI) (2003) *Clinical Trials – Developing New Medicines*. ABPI, London.

Audit Commission (2002) *Setting the Record Straight*. Audit Commission, London.

Bolam v *Friern HMC* [1957] 1 WLR 582.

Brindley M (2003) Doctors find code writing is best way to treat patients. *The Western Mail*, p. 8, 19th August.

Collins v *Hertfordshire County Council* (1947) KB 598.

Council Directive (EC) 2001/20 (2001) on the approximation of the laws, regulations and administrative provisions of the Member States relating to implementation of good clinical practice in the conduct of clinical trials on medicinal products for human use. OJ L121/34.

Deacon v *McVicar* (1984) (Unreported Queens Bench Division, 7th June).

Department for Constitutional Affairs (2007) *Mental Capacity Act 2005 Code of Practice*. The Stationery Office, London.

Department of Health (DH) (2003) *An Organisation with a Memory*. DH, London.

Department of Health (DH) (2005) *Supplementary Prescribing by Nurses, Pharmacists, Chiropodists/Podiatrists, Physiotherapists and Radiographers within the NHS in England: a Guide for Implementation*. DH, London.

Dwyer v *Rodrick* (1983) 80 LSG 3003.

Gerber v *Pines* (1939) 79 SJ 13.

Goorkani v *Tayside Health Board* [1991] SLT 94.

Horler v *Kingston and Esher Health Authority* [1993] EWHC 361.

Jordan S, Griffiths H, Griffith RA (2003) Administration of medicines part 2: pharmacology. *Nurs Stand* **18**(3): 45–54.

Kent v *Griffiths & Others* [2000] 3 CLL Rep 98.

Marriott v *West Midlands HA* [1999] Lloyd's Rep Med 23.

Marsh B, Narain J (2003) Patient died because of GP's bad handwriting (news item). *Daily Mail*, p. 4, 4th February.

McLennan v *Newcastle HA* [1992] 3 Med LR 215.

Medicines and Healthcare products Regulatory Agency (MHRA) (2003) *Supplementary Prescribing*. MHRA, London.

Medicines for Human Use (Clinical Trials) Regulations 2004 (SI 2004/1031).

Medicines for Human Use (Prescribing) (Miscellaneous Amendments) Order 2006 (SI 2006/915).

Misuse of Drugs (Amendment) Regulations 2005.

Misuse of Drugs Regulations 2001 (SI 2001/3998).

Nash v *Eli Lilley* [1993] 1 WLR 782.

National Health Service (General Medical Services Contracts) (Personal Medical Services Agreements) and (Pharmaceutical Services) (Amendment) Regulations 2005.

National Patient Safety Agency (NPSA) (2007) *The Fourth Report from the Patient Safety Observatory. Safety in Doses: Medication Safety Incidents in the NHS*. The Stationery Office, London.

National Prescribing Centre (2004) *Patient Group Directions: a Practical Guide and Framework of Competencies for All Professionals Using Patient Group Directions*. National Prescribing Centre, London.

NHS Litigation Authority (2007) *Report and Accounts 2007 (HC 908)*. The Stationery Office, London.

Nurse struck off for stealing medicines (2008) *Western Mail News*, p. 10, February 5th.

Nursing & Midwifery Council (NMC) (2002) *Cardiff Nurse Struck off over Patient Abuse; NMC Press Statement 184/02*. NMC, London.

Nursing & Midwifery Council (NMC) (2003) *Nurse Cautioned About Prescribing Without Qualification – NMC Press Release 390*. NMC, London.

Nursing & Midwifery Council (NMC) (2006) *Standards of Proficiency for Nurse and Midwife Prescribers*. NMC, London.

Nursing & Midwifery Council (NMC) (2007a) *Covert Administration of Medicines – Advice Sheet*. NMC, London.

Nursing & Midwifery Council (NMC) (2007b) *Crushing Tablets – NMC Advice Sheet*. NMC, London.

Nursing & Midwifery Council (NMC) (2008a) *The Code: Standards of Conduct, Performance and Ethics for Nurses and Midwives*. NMC, London.

Nursing & Midwifery Council (NMC) (2008b) *Fitness to Practise Annual Report 2007–08*. NMC, London.

Nursing & Midwifery Council (NMC) (2008c) *Standards for Medicines Management*. NMC, London.

Nursing & Midwifery Order 2001 (SI 2002/253).

Pirmohamed M, James S, Meakin S, *et al.* (2004) Adverse drug reactions as a cause of admission to hospital: prospective analysis of 18 820 patients. *BMJ* **329**: 15–19.

Prendergast v *Sam and Dee* (1989) 1 Med LR 36.

Prescription Only Medicines (Human Use) Order 1997 (SI 1997/1830).

Pretty v *DPP* [2001] UKHL 61.

R v *Cox* (1992) 12 BMLR 38.

R v *Moor* (2000) Crim LR 41.

R v *Salisbury* [2005] EWCA Crim 3107 (CA).

R v *Shipman* [2000] (Crown Ct) (Unreported).

Re T (Adult: Refusal of Treatment) [1992] 3 WLR.

Re W (A Minor) (Medical Treatment: Court's Jurisdiction) [1993] Fam 64 (CA).

Reynolds v *North Tyneside Health Authority* [2002] Lloyd's Rep Med 459.

S v *Distillers Co (Biochemicals) Ltd* [1970] 1 WLR 114.

S (A Child) v *Newcastle & North Tyneside HA* [2001] EWCA Civ 1868.

Saunders v *Leeds Western HA* [1993] 4 Med LR 355.

Smith v *Brighton and Lewes Hospital Management Committee* (1958). Times Law Report, 2 May.

Strokes P (2005) GP cleared of three murders faces 12 further inquiries. *Telegraph*, g 3, 16th December.

The Mental Capacity Act 2005 (Independent Mental Capacity Advocate) (General) Regulations 2006 (2006/1832).

The Shipman Inquiry (2004a) *Fifth Report: Safeguarding Patients: Lessons from the Past – Proposals for the Future (Cm 6394).* The Stationery Office, London.

The Shipman Inquiry (2004b) *Fourth Report: The Regulation of Controlled Drugs in the Community (Cm 6249).* The Stationery Office, London.

Whitehouse v *Jordan* (1981) 1 All ER 267 (HL).

Safety in Medicines Management

3

Elizabeth Payne

INTRODUCTION

Legislation plays an important role in safeguarding healthcare professionals and patients from the potential hazards involved in handling all manner of substances that healthcare professionals come into contact when caring for patients, such as body fluids, chemicals, medicines and equipments.

The Health and Safety at Work etc Act 1974 places a legal duty on employers to provide for the health and safety of their employees. NHS organisations have been subject to the full requirements of this legislation since 1991. These duties were extended under the Management of Health and Safety at Work Regulations 1992, which require employers to:

- assess risks to the health and safety of their employees;
- arrange for implementing a comprehensive system of safety management.

By failing to prevent injuries, NHS organisations can be found in breach of health and safety regulations, which can result in substantial legal expenses and compensation payments.

Under the Control of Substances Hazardous to Health (COSHH) Regulations 2002 [Health and Safety Executive (2009)], the law requires employers to make a suitable and sufficient assessment of the risks to the health of workers exposed to such substances, with a view to preventing or adequately controlling the risks. This includes the proper use of protective equipment and regular monitoring of exposure.

These regulations are pivotal to ensuring that a healthcare worker's work environment does not cause ill health. In the light of this, a proportion of this chapter is devoted to exploring what is required by COSHH.

More recently, with the Health Act 2006, the emphasis has focused on re-establishing the duty of care the NHS has towards protecting patients from potential hazards. Hence, another section of this chapter looks at universal precautions and safe waste disposal practice. Expanding on this theme, it is also pertinent to consider the safe handling of medicines and the mechanism whereby adverse drug reactions (ADRs) are reported.

The aim of this chapter is to understand safety in medicines management.

LEARNING OUTCOMES

At the end of this chapter, the reader will be able to:

❑ Discuss Control of Substances Hazardous to Health Regulations.
❑ Outline universal infection control precautions.
❑ Discuss the principles of waste disposal.
❑ Describe the principles of safe handling of medicines.
❑ Discuss the procedure for reporting an adverse drug reaction.

CONTROL OF SUBSTANCES HAZARDOUS TO HEALTH

COSHH Regulations

COSHH Regulations specifically require the employer to:

- identify hazardous substances and practices;
- assess risks to exposure to hazardous substances in the workplace, and if significant:
  ○ provide a safe working environment through control of exposure to the hazardous substances;
  ○ monitor and maintain a safe working environment where hazardous substances are used.

Hazardous substances

Hazardous substances include:

- substances used directly in work activities (e.g. adhesives, paints and cleaning agents);

- substances generated during work activities (e.g. fumes from soldering and welding);
- naturally occurring substances (e.g. grain dust);
- biological agents such as bacteria and other micro-organisms.

For the vast majority of commercial chemicals, the presence (or not) of a hazard warning label will indicate whether COSHH is relevant. For example, there is no warning label on ordinary household washing-up liquid, so if it is used at work then it is not necessary to apply COSHH. On the other hand, household bleach does contain a hazard warning label, and so if it is used at work COSHH Regulations apply.

Examples of hazard warning labels are shown in Figure 3.1.

Many dangerous substances are listed in the Health and Safety Executive's (HSE) *The Approved Supply List*. However, even if the substance is not listed in *The Approved Supply List* but the supplier of a substance believes the substance to be dangerous, hazard warning labelling and a material safety data sheet should be provided.

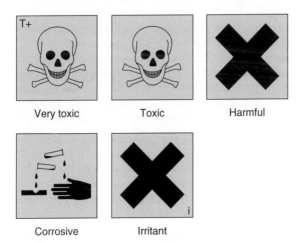

Fig 3.1 Examples of hazard warning labels. Reproduced under the terms of the click-use licence

COSHH applies to virtually all substances hazardous to health except:

- asbestos and lead, which have their own regulations;
- substances that are hazardous only because they are:
  - radioactive;
  - asphyxiants;
  - used at high pressure and/or extreme temperatures;
  - have explosive or flammable properties (other regulations apply to these risks);
- biological agents that are outside the employer's control, e.g. catching an infection from a workmate.

Effects of exposure to hazardous substances

Exposure to a substance can occur via inhalation, absorption, ingestion or injection. Uncontrolled exposure to hazardous substances can cause:

- irritation of the skin, dermatitis and cancers;
- asthma and other breathing impairments (e.g. asbestosis) arising from cumulative sensitisation and dusts, asphyxia, or poisoning by toxic fumes, including smoking-mediated reactions;
- cancers that typically appear years after initial exposure to cancer-causing (carcinogenic) substances;
- poisoning or burning by transferring noxious substances to the mouth by unwashed hands or by consuming from wrongly labelled bottles (e.g. acids in originally labelled soft-drink bottles), overdosing on medicines and through an open wound;
- infection from bacteria and other micro-organisms.

Hence, if an exposure to a hazardous substance is not properly controlled or prevented, it can cause serious illness, resulting in lost income for the individual and reduced productivity as well as the possibility of expensive prosecution and litigation for a business. Uncontrolled exposure can ultimately cause the death of an individual and closure of the business.

Key requirements of COSHH

To comply with COSHH, an employer must follow eight steps as follows:

Step 1: Assess the risks

Firstly, identify the hazardous substances present in the work-place or created by workplace activities.

Secondly, consider the risks these substances present to people's health. This is known as a risk assessment and the following questions should be asked:

- How much of the substance is in use or produced by the work activity and how could people be exposed to it?
- Who could be exposed to the substance and how often?
- Is there a possibility of substances being absorbed through the skin or swallowed (e.g. as a result of a substance getting into the mouth from contaminated hands during eating or smoking)?
- Are there risks to employees at other locations if they work away from their main workplace?

Step 2: Decide what precautions are needed

Decide on the action needed to remove identified risks or reduce them to acceptable levels. Any controls already in place should be compared with the information contained in *COSHH essentials; easy steps to control chemicals*, workplace exposure limits (WELs) published in *EH40/2005 Workplace exposure limits*, good work practices, and standards used by or recommended for the particular employment sector, e.g. Health and Safety Commission (HSC) advisory committees. If there is no risk to health or the risk is trivial, then the identity of the substance, the control measures taken, and the fact that it poses little or no risk should be recorded. If risks to health are subsequently identified, the employer must take action to protect its employees' health by following the eight steps described.

A record should be made as soon as practicable after a risk assessment has been done and contain enough information to explain the decisions taken about whether risks are significant and the need for any control measures. The actions employees and others need to take to ensure that hazardous substances are adequately controlled should also be recorded. The risk assessment should be a 'living' document, which is reviewed whenever circumstances change; the assessment should state when the next review is planned and be available for viewing by health and safety inspectors.

Step 3: Prevent or adequately control exposure

To prevent exposure the employer may need to:

- change the process or activity so that the hazardous substance is not needed or generated;
- replace the process or activity with a safer alternative;
- use the process or activity in a safer form, e.g. pellets instead of powder.

If prevention is practicable, the employer must put in place measures appropriate to the activity and consistent with the risk assessment in order to adequately control exposure, such as one or more of the following, in order of priority:

- Use appropriate work processes, systems and engineering controls, and suitable work equipment and materials, e.g. processes that minimise the amount of material used or produced, or equipment that totally encloses the process.
- Control exposure at source (e.g. local exhaust ventilation) and reduce the number of employees exposed to a minimum, the level and duration of their exposure, and the quantity of hazardous substances used or produced in the workplace.
- Provide personal protective equipment (PPE) (e.g. face masks, respirators and protective clothing), but only as a last resort and never as a replacement for other required control measures.

Under COSHH, adequate control of exposure to a substance hazardous to health means:

- applying the eight steps described;
- not exceeding the WEL (a WEL is the maximum concentration of an airborne substance, averaged over a reference period, to which employees may be exposed by inhalation and is intended to prevent excessive exposure to specified hazardous substances by containing exposure below a set limit) for the substance (if there is one);

- reducing exposure to as low a level as is reasonably practicable if the substance causes cancer, heritable genetic damage or asthma.

Step 4: Ensure that control measures are used and maintained

COSHH requires employees to make proper use of control measures and to report defects, but the employer must have taken all reasonable steps to ensure that they do so.

COSHH places specific duties on the employer to ensure that exposure controls are maintained so that every element of the control measure performs as intended. This applies to items of equipment such as local exhaust ventilation, and to systems of work, which will have to be regularly checked to make sure that they are still effective, for example respiratory protective equipment and local ventilation equipment should be tested at suitable intervals. COSHH sets specific intervals between examinations for the latter, and the employer must retain records of examinations and tests carried out (or a summary of them) for at least 5 years.

Step 5: Monitor the exposure

The concentration of hazardous substances in the air breathed in by employees must be measured where an assessment concludes that:

- there could be serious risks to health if control measures failed or deteriorated;
- exposure limits might be exceeded;
- control measures might not be working properly.

The above is not required if another method of evaluation demonstrates that employees' exposure to hazardous substances is prevented or adequately controlled, e.g. a system that automatically sounds an alarm if it detects hazardous substances.

Air monitoring should be carried out when employees are exposed to certain substances and processes specified in Schedule 5 of the COSHH Regulations.

A record of any exposure monitoring carried out for at least 5 years must be saved and maintained. Where employees have a health record (required where they are under health surveillance, see Step 6), any monitoring results relevant to them as individuals must be kept with their health records. They should be allowed access to their personal monitoring records.

Step 6: Carry out appropriate health surveillance

Health surveillance must be carried out in the following circumstances:

- where an employee is exposed to one of the substances listed in Schedule 6 of COSHH and is working in one of the related processes, e.g. manufacture of certain compounds of benzene, *and* there is a reasonable likelihood that an identifiable disease or adverse health effect will result from that exposure;
- where an employee is exposed to a substance linked to a particular disease or an adverse health effect *and* there is a reasonable likelihood, under the conditions of the work, of that disease or effect occurring *and* it is possible to detect the disease or health effect.

Step 7: Prepare plans and procedures to deal with accidents, incidents and emergencies

Standard operating procedures and warning and communication systems must be put in place to enable an appropriate response immediately any incident occurs. Information on emergency arrangements should be available to those who need to see it, including the emergency services. Safety drills should be practised at regular intervals.

If any accident, incident or emergency occurs, immediate steps should be taken to minimise the harmful effects, restore the situation to normal and inform employees who may be affected. Only those staff necessary to deal with the incident should remain in the area and they must be provided with appropriate safety equipment.

These emergency procedures are not required if:

- the quantities of substances hazardous to health present in the workplace are such that they present only a slight risk to employees' health;

- the measures put in place under Step 3 are sufficient to control that risk.

However, the requirements described in Step 7 should be complied with in full where carcinogens, mutagens or biological agents are used.

Step 8: Ensure employees are properly informed, trained and supervised

The employer must provide employees with suitable and sufficient information, instruction and training, which should include:

- the names of the substances they work with or could be exposed to and the risks created by such exposure, and access to any safety data sheets that apply to those substances;
- the main findings of any risk assessment;
- the precautions employees should take to protect themselves and other employees;
- how to use PPE and clothing provided;
- results of any exposure monitoring and health surveillance (without giving individual employees' names);
- emergency procedures that need to be followed.

The information, instruction and training should be updated and adapted to take account of significant changes in the type of work or work methods used. Information should be provided that is appropriate to the level of risk identified by the assessment and is easily understood by employees.

UNIVERSAL INFECTION CONTROL PRECAUTIONS

'Universal precautions' were first recommended by the Centers for Disease Control in America (1987), in response to the risk of transmission of human immunodeficiency virus (HIV) to healthcare workers from patients whose infection status was unknown. Initially they dealt only with body fluids capable of containing blood-borne viruses such as the hepatitis B and C viruses (HBV and HCV), but the concept was later expanded to include all body substances capable of containing pathogenic micro-organisms, which could potentially lead to cross-infection between patients. This expanded version is known as 'universal infection control precautions'. Some hospitals use the term 'universal infection control precautions' (UICPs) and others use 'standard precautions'. These terms are now interchangeable.

UICPs are based on a risk assessment of the likelihood of exposure to blood, all body fluids, secretions and excretions except sweat, regardless of whether or not they contain visible blood, non-intact skin and mucous membranes, and not on an assessment of the perceived risk of infection from the individual patient. Many patients who carry pathogens may not be aware of this fact, or they may choose not to disclose it to their carers. By adopting UICPs, the risk of transmission of pathogens is minimised from these patients. This approach also means a non-discriminatory approach to patients known to carry or suspected of carrying pathogens. Use of UICPs reduces the risk of transmission of pathogens from both recognised and unrecognised sources of infection.

The National Institute for Clinical Excellence [National Institute for Clinical Excellence (NICE), 2003] produced clinical guidelines for the prevention of healthcare-associated infections (HCAI) in primary and community care based on the best critically appraised evidence available. Subsequently, the Government produced a new and specific code of practice encapsulated in the Health Act 2006, which puts a statutory duty on NHS healthcare organisations to protect patients, staff and other persons against the risks of acquiring HCAI through the provision of appropriate care, in suitable facilities, consistent with good clinical practice [Department of Health (DH), 2006a].

Hence, UICPs are essential for delivering the outcomes required by good practice and legislation and consist of the following measures.

Hand decontamination

In September 2004, the National Patient Safety Agency [National Patient Safety Agency (NPSA), 2004, updated 2008] issued a patient safety alert advising all NHS organisations to install alcohol-based hand rubs at points of patient care. At the same time, the NPSA launched a national 'clean*your*hands' campaign that aimed to increase hand hygiene compliance amongst healthcare professionals and reduce the human and financial burden of HCAI. The campaign is multi-modal and evidence based, and consists of a toolkit of products and recommended methods to facilitate improvement in hand hygiene compliance. The toolkit reinforces the need for the standard provision of alcohol-based hand rub (either at each bedside or to each caregiver). The products include posters and promotional messages designed to act as psychological prompts to healthcare professionals and information for the empowerment of patients in the hand hygiene process.

The World Health Organization [World Health Organization (WHO), 2009] guidelines on hand hygiene in health care have conducted a comprehensive literature review on the burden of HCAI worldwide and have cited hand hygiene as one of the most effective measures in reducing and preventing the incidence of avoidable illness, in particular HCAI.

The following are recommendations drawn from NICE and WHO guidance:

- All wrist and, ideally, hand jewellery should be removed before regular hand decontamination begins. Cuts and abrasions should be covered with waterproof dressings. Fingernails should be kept short (tips less than 0.5 cm long), clean and free from nail polish; artificial nails or extenders should not be worn.
- Hand hygiene should be carried out:
  ○ before and after having direct contact with patients;
  ○ after removing gloves;
  ○ before handling an invasive device for patient care, regardless of whether or not gloves are used;
  ○ after contact with body fluids or excretions, mucous membranes, non-intact skin or wound dressings;
  ○ if moving from a contaminated body site to a clean body site during patient care;
  ○ after contact with inanimate objects (including medical equipment) in the immediate vicinity of the patient.
  Hands that are visibly soiled, or potentially grossly contaminated with dirt or organic material, should be washed with liquid soap and water. Otherwise hands should be decontaminated with an alcohol-based hand rub.

- An effective handwashing technique involves three stages: preparation, washing and rinsing, and drying. Preparation requires wetting hands under tepid running water before applying liquid soap or an antimicrobial preparation. The handwash solution must come into contact with all of the surfaces of the hand. The hands must be rubbed together vigorously for a minimum of 10–15 seconds, paying particular attention to the tips of the fingers, the thumbs and the areas between the fingers. Hands should be rinsed thoroughly before drying with good quality paper towels.
- When decontaminating hands using an alcohol hand rub, hands should be free from dirt and organic material. The hand-rub solution should come into contact with all surfaces of the hand. The hands should be *rubbed* together vigorously, paying particular attention to the tips of the fingers, the thumbs and the areas between the fingers, until the solution has evaporated and the hands are dry.
- An emollient hand cream should be applied regularly to protect skin from the drying effects of regular hand decontamination. If a particular soap, antimicrobial hand wash or alcohol product causes skin irritation, an occupational health team should be consulted.

Personal protective equipment

Over the past 20 years there has been a trend to eliminate the inappropriate wearing of aprons, gowns and masks in general care settings because of a lack of evidence that they are effective in preventing HCAI. Hence, the decision to use or wear PPE should be based on an assessment of the risk of transmission of micro-organisms to the patient, the risk of contamination of the healthcare professional's clothing and skin by patients' blood, body fluids, secretions or excretions, and take account of current health and safety legislation.

The following recommendations are drawn from NICE and WHO guidance:

- Gloves should be worn for invasive procedures, contact with sterile sites and non-intact skin or mucous membranes, and all activities that have been assessed as carrying a risk of exposure to blood, body fluids, secretions or excretions, or to sharp or contaminated instruments. They should be worn as single-use items, put on immediately before an episode of patient contact or treatment and removed as soon as the activity is completed. Gloves should be changed between caring for different patients, and between different care or treatment activities for the same patient, and should be disposed of as clinical waste.

- Gloves that conform to European Community (CE) standards should be available. Sensitivity to natural rubber latex in patients, carers and healthcare personnel should be documented, and alternatives to natural rubber latex gloves should be available. Neither powdered gloves nor polythene gloves should be used in healthcare activities.
- Disposable plastic aprons should be worn when there is a risk that clothing may be exposed to blood, body'fluids, secretions or excretions, with the exception of sweat. These should be worn as single-use items then discarded and disposed of as clinical waste, following a procedure or episode of patient care. Full-body fluid-repellent gowns should be worn where there is a risk of extensive splashing of blood, body fluids, secretions or excretions, with the exception of sweat, onto the skin or clothing of healthcare practitioners (for example when assisting with childbirth).
- Face masks and eye protection should be worn where there is a risk of blood, body fluids, secretions or excretions splashing into the face and eyes. Respiratory protective equipment, such as a particulate filter mask, should be used when clinically indicated.

Safe sharps use and disposal

Of the occupational injuries that occur in hospitals, 16% are attributable to sharps injuries.

A sharps or needlestick injury (NSI) can be defined as an injury from a needle or any other device that has been contaminated with blood or other body fluid and penetrates the skin percutaneously (superficially).

A 7-year study conducted by the Health Protection Agency (HPA) entitled *Eye of the Needle* (HPA, 2008) published data collated across 150 reporting centres on significant occupational exposure to blood-borne viruses amongst healthcare workers.

The study reported that NSIs were the most commonly reported type of significant exposure, with 68% of those injuries caused by hollow bore needles. Just under a half of these occurred amongst nursing professionals and around a third amongst medical professionals. A much lower incidence was identified amongst professions allied to medicine and ancillary staff. Only 2% of the exposures occurred in ancillary staff, but most were sustained from inappropriately discarded needles in rubbish bags. In the 7-year period covered by the study, there were 14 documented seroconversions (positive immune responses) for HCV virus, five seroconversions for HIV and no seroconversions for HBV virus.

The average risk of transmission of blood-borne pathogens following a single percutaneous exposure from a positive source has been estimated to be:

- HBV 33.3% (1 in 3);
- HCV 3.3% (1 in 30);
- HIV 0.31% (1 in 319).

NSIs are predominantly avoidable, and any reduction in NSIs is primarily dependent on high-quality education and training, and effective monitoring and audit. The employer is obliged to provide local protocols and information on the risk of blood-borne viruses in the work place and to ensure that healthcare workers are adequately trained on how to prevent injuries. A national blended e-learning programme on preventing HCAI is available for all healthcare workers at www.infectioncontrol.nhs. uk. In addition, the Centers for Disease Control and Prevention has developed an online programme focused on implementing and evaluating a sharps injury prevention programme at www. cdc.gov/sharpssafety.

National and international guidelines are consistent in their recommendations for the safe use and disposal of sharp instruments and needles (DH, 1998; Centers for Disease Control, 1999). As with many infection prevention and control policies, the assessment and management of the risks associated with the use of sharps is paramount, and safe systems of work and engineering controls must be in place to minimise any identified risks, e.g. positioning the sharps bin as close as possible to the site of the intended clinical procedure.

The following summarises the safety precautions that should be observed when using and disposing of sharps:

- Locate sharps containers in a safe position, not on the floor.
- Do not pass sharps directly from hand to hand, keep handling to a minimum.
- Avoid recapping, bending, breaking or disassembling used needles.
- Use a sharps box with a needle-removing facility if removal of the needle from the syringe is unavoidable or use forceps or approach the needle carefully along the barrel of the syringe, using a gloved hand, taking extreme care.
- Discard disposable sharps in an appropriate sharps container (see below) situated at the point of use.
- Do not overfill the container.
- Drop items in carefully; do not push items down.
- Dispose of containers by the licensed route, according to local policy.
- Consider the use of needle safety devices where there are clear indications that they will provide safer systems of working for healthcare workers.

Sharps containers should comply with British Standard 7320, United Nations Standard 3291 or their equivalent. Sharps containers must:

- be puncture resistant and leak proof, even if they fall over or are dropped;
- be capable of being handled and moved whilst in use;
- have a handle that is not part of the closure device and does not interfere with the normal use of the container;
- have an opening that, in normal use, will inhibit removal of contents but allow disposal of items with one hand, without contaminating the outside of the container;
- have a closure device attached for sealing when the container is three-quarters full or ready for disposal;
- have a horizontal line to indicate when the container is three-quarters full and be marked with the words 'Warning – do not fill above the line';

- be made of material that can be incinerated;
- be yellow;
- be clearly marked with the words 'Danger', 'Contaminated sharps' and 'Destroy by incineration' or 'To be incinerated'.

PRINCIPLES OF WASTE DISPOSAL

Clinical waste, as defined in the Controlled Waste Regulations 1992, means any waste that consists wholly or partly of:

- human or animal tissue;
- blood or bodily fluids;
- excretions;
- drugs or other pharmaceutical products;
- swabs or dressings;
- syringes, needles or other sharp instruments;

which unless rendered safe may prove hazardous to any person coming into contact with it, and:

- any other waste arising from medical, nursing, dental, veterinary, pharmaceutical or similar practice, investigation, treatment, care, teaching or research, or the collection of blood for transfusion, being waste which may cause infection to any person coming into contact with it.

The Department of Health (DH, 2006b) published a health technical memorandum on the safe management of healthcare waste on 1 December 2006. This provides a best practice guide and takes into account the legislation governing the management of waste, its storage, carriage, treatment and disposal, and health and safety (www.dh.gov.uk/en/Publicationsandstatistics/Publications/PublicationsPolicyAndGuidance/DH_063274).

The main focus of the above-named document is the segregation of waste at the point of production into suitable colour-coded packaging, which is considered vital to good waste management. The colour-coded segregation system identifies and segregates waste on the basis of waste classification and suitability of treatment/disposal options. The use of this colour-coding system is not mandatory and is not specified in regulations.

The charts in the above-named document identify the type of packaging and packaging colour required for each waste stream.

The charts assume that the packaging meets the requirements of the Carriage Regulations (UN compliant) where appropriate.

Historically there has been limited segregation of waste. However, the recent changes to the Hazardous Waste Regulations mean that there is now a greater emphasis on waste minimisation in the healthcare sector, with the segregation of non-infectious waste from infectious waste, assuming a higher priority and a policy of 'reduce, reuse and recycle' being employed wherever possible and practical. Since 2002, co-disposal of hazardous and non-hazardous waste is no longer allowed. Complying with new legislation and guidelines on reducing landfill and the safe disposal of hospital waste is an increasingly complex and expensive business, so it is vitally important that healthcare professionals think about what they throw away and where.

The waste industry is heavily regulated by EU directives, Acts of Parliament, departmental guidelines, Secretary of State Regulations and Environment Agency Codes of Practice. Failure to comply with all these regulations carries potentially heavy penalties. The Magistrates Court can impose prison sentences of up to a year and fines up to £50 000. The Crown Court can impose unlimited fines and prison terms of up to 5 years.

PRINCIPLES OF SAFE HANDLING OF MEDICINES

The term 'medicines' embraces all products that are administered by mouth, applied to the body or introduced into the body for the purpose of treating or preventing disease, diagnosing disease, ascertaining the existence, degree or extent of a physiological condition, contraception, inducing anaesthesia, or otherwise preventing or interfering with the normal operation of a physiological function.

There is relatively little legislation concerning the handling of medicines within the NHS. Key legislation includes the Medicines Act 1968, the Misuse of Drugs Act 1971 and its associated regulations, the Prescription-Only Medicines (human use) Order 1997, the Health Act 2006, the Controlled Drugs (Supervision of Management and use) Regulations 2006, the Health and Safety at Work etc Act, the Control of Substances Hazardous to Health Regulations 2002 and the Hazardous Waste Regulations 2005.

There have been a number of publications focusing on the safe and secure handling of medicines within the NHS since it was first established in 1948: the Aitken report (1958), the Annis–Gillie report (1970), the Roxburgh report (1972), the Duthie report (1988) and *The Safe and Secure Handling of Medicines: a Team Approach* [Royal Pharmaceutical Society of Great Britain (RPSGB), 2005]. These publications have each in turn filled in the gaps between legislation and NHS guidance, and have been used to support professional practice and underpin medicines risk management.

There have been a number of key changes over the last two decades that have influenced the safe handling of medicines:

- Increasing emphasis on good clinical governance. Clinical governance is the system through which NHS organisations are accountable for continuously improving the quality of their services and safeguarding high standards of care, by creating an environment in which clinical excellence will flourish.
- Growing awareness of medication errors, which has led to the establishment of the NPSA.
- Growth in public expectations that their treatments will meet the highest of standards.
- Changing models of patient care such as reduced hospital stay, increase in day case procedures, development of medical support units away from hospitals, growth of treatment at home, self-administration of medicines in hospital, continued use of patient's own medicines whilst in hospital and dispensing for discharge – so-called 'one-stop' dispensing.
- Technological advances such as computerised prescribing, automated dispensing, electronic recording of administration and rapid, economic procurement of medicines as well as rapid transfer of information between primary and secondary care and vice versa.
- The developing roles of healthcare staff, such as non-medical prescribing.

PROCEDURE FOR REPORTING AN ADR

The guidance to reporting ADRs described in this section is based on that published by the British Medical Association (BMA, 2006).

Definition of an ADR

The Medicines and Healthcare products Regulatory Agency (MHRA) defines an ADR as 'an unwanted or harmful reaction experienced following the administration of a drug or combination of drugs, and is suspected to be related to the drug. The reaction may be a known side effect of the drug or it may be new and previously unrecognised'. This is different to an adverse event, which is 'any undesirable experience that has happened to the patient while taking a drug but may or may not be related to the drug'.

The MHRA provides guidance on factors that should be considered when trying to establish the cause of a reaction on their website at www.mhra.gov.uk such as, for example, the nature of the reaction, the timing of the reaction in relation to drug administration, the relationship to the dose administered and other possible causes of the reaction, including concomitant medications and the patient's underlying disease.

Frequency of ADRs

It is difficult to identify an ADR because it varies in its severity, in the nature of the drug that caused the ADR and in what setting the ADR occurred. It is therefore virtually impossible to determine the exact number of ADRs that occur because of the difficulty in finding out the cause and because so few ADRs are reported.

The majority of research that has tried to quantify ADRs has done so by evaluating hospital patients, particularly admissions. A study of hospital admissions in the UK, published in 2004, found that 6.5% of people admitted to hospital had experienced an ADR and that, in 80% of these cases, the ADR was the reason for the admission. This research (which excluded admissions due to drug overdose) also found that ADRs accounted for 4% of hospital bed capacity and resulted in a projected annual cost to the NHS of £466m. There has been little research into the incidence of ADRs in patients treated in primary care. One small study in the USA found that around 25% of outpatients had experienced an ADR and that in many instances they were preventable.

Importance of reporting ADRs

Little may be known about the safety of a medicine when it is first marketed. This is because during clinical trials, when a medicine is going through preliminary tests before it is licensed, only a small number of patients, who are relatively healthy with only one disease (not pregnant women, children and the elderly), are exposed to the medicine over a limited period of time, compared to the number of patients who might use it once it is licensed. Rare ADRs that occur in only a small percentage of cases, after a long period of use or when a drug interacts with a particular combination of other medications or conditions are unlikely to be detected during clinical trials. Thus, it is essential that once a medicine has been licensed and marketed surveillance is carried out in order to identify medicine safety problems not picked up by pre-marketing tests. Furthermore, it is essential to communicate any necessary advice and/or regulatory action to prescribers and users subsequent to identifying medicine safety problems. ADR reporting, whether spontaneous, from pharmaceutical manufacturers, from patient mortality/morbidity databases or published medical literature, is used to generate hypotheses about the potential hazards of marketed medicines that require further investigation. Spontaneous reporting of suspected ADRs is particularly useful in identifying rare or delayed reactions; such a system enables medicines to be monitored throughout their lifetime. Databases containing patient or prescription data reflect the routine usage of medications in the general population and provide baseline data, which can be used to identify trends and so lead to improvements in patient care.

How to report an ADR

In the UK, a voluntary, spontaneous reporting scheme, the Yellow Card Scheme (Figure 3.2), run by the MHRA and the Commission on Human Medicines (CHM), is used to collect information on ADRs. The Yellow Card Scheme relies on the goodwill of reporters; healthcare professionals should consider it their professional duty to report ADRs. Since the original CHM, known as the Committee on Safety of Drugs, was established in 1964 following the thalidomide tragedy, over half a million reports have been

Yellowcard

In Confidence

MHRA

COMMISSION ON
HUMAN MEDICINES

SUSPECTED ADVERSE DRUG REACTIONS

If you suspect that an adverse reaction may be related to a drug, or a combination of drugs, you should complete this Yellow Card or complete a report on the website at www.yellowcard.gov.uk. For *intensively monitored medicines* (identified by ▼) report **all** suspected reactions (including any considered not to be serious). For *established drugs* and *herbal remedies* report **all serious** adverse reactions in adults; report **all serious and minor** adverse reactions in **children** (under 18 years). You do not have to be certain about causality: if in doubt, please report. Do not be put off reporting just because some details are not known. See BNF (page 11) or the MHRA website (www.yellowcard.gov.uk) for additional advice.

PATIENT DETAILS   Patient Initials: _____   Sex: M / F   Weight if known (kg): _____

Age (at time of reaction): _____   Identification (Your Practice / Hospital Ref.)*: _____

SUSPECTED DRUG(S)

Give brand name of drug and batch number if known	Route	Dosage	Date started	Date stopped	Prescribed for

Outcome

Recovered ☐☐☐☐
Recovering
Continuing
Other ☐☐

SUSPECTED REACTION(S)
Please describe the reaction(s) and any treatment given:

Date reaction(s) started: _____   Date reaction(s) stopped: _____

Do you consider the reaction to be serious? Yes / No

If yes, please indicate why the reaction is considered to be serious (please tick all that apply):

Patient died due to reaction ☐   Involved or prolonged inpatient hospitalisation
Life threatening ☐   Involved persistent or significant disability or incapacity
Congenital abnormality ☐   Medically significant; please give details:

* This is to enable you to identify the patient in any future correspondence concerning this report

Fig 3.2 Yellow Card Scheme for reporting a suspected ADR. Reproduced with permission of the MHRA

Please attach additional pages if necessary

Please list other drugs taken in the last 3 months prior to the reaction (including self-medication & herbal remedies)

Was the patient on any other medication?   Yes / No   If yes, please give the following information if known:

Drug (Brand, if known)	Route	Dosage	Date started	Date stopped	Prescribed for

Additional relevant information e.g. medical history, test results, known allergies, rechallenge (if performed), suspected drug interactions. For congenital abnormalities please state all other drugs taken during pregnancy and the date of the last menstrual period.

REPORTER DETAILS
Name and Professional Address:

Post code: Tel No:
Speciality:
Signature: Date:

CLINICIAN (if not the reporter)
Name and Professional Address:

                         Post code:
Tel No: Speciality:

If you would like information about other adverse reactions associated with the suspected drug, please tick this box   ☐

If you report from an area served by a Yellow Card Centre (YCC), MHRA may ask the Centre to communicate with you, on its behalf, about your report. See BNF (page 11) for further details on YCCs. If you want only MHRA to contact you, please tick this box.   ☐

Send to **Medicines and Healthcare products Regulatory Agency, CHM FREEPOST, LONDON SW8 5BR**

Fig 3.2 *Continued*

collected. Detailed information about the Yellow Card Scheme can be found on the MHRA website at www.mhra.gov.uk.

Originally only medical and dental prescribers could submit reports. This has gradually been extended, and now all healthcare professionals, including coroners, pharmacists and nurses, are able to report ADRs via the scheme. Furthermore, patients may now report any ADRs they experience directly. The database used by the MHRA can detect duplicate reports and therefore a healthcare professional should submit a Yellow Card regardless of whether or not someone else might have reported the same ADR. Different people will include different information when they complete a Yellow Card, all of which is useful in creating a full picture of the reaction that has taken place. Yellow Cards should be submitted to either the MHRA or to one of five regional monitoring centres (RMC). Paper Yellow Cards are available by writing to either the MHRA or one of the RMCs, and can also be found in copies of the BNF, the Nurse Prescribers' Formulary (NPF), the Monthly Index of Medical Specialties (MIMS) Companion and from the Association of the British Pharmaceutical Industry (ABPI) Compendium of Data Sheets and Summaries of Product Characteristics. Electronic Yellow Cards were introduced in 2002 and can be downloaded from either the MHRA or the RMC websites (www.yellowcard.gov.uk). The MHRA also receives ADR reports from pharmaceutical companies, which have a statutory obligation to report suspected serious ADRs. If a healthcare professional passes details of an ADR on to the pharmaceutical firm that markets the drug, this information will subsequently be passed on to the MHRA.

What should be reported via the Yellow Card Scheme

In the BNF it is noted that an ADR can be caused by any therapeutic agent, including prescribed and over-the-counter (OTC) drugs, blood products, vaccines, radiographic contrast media and herbal products, and that all of these should be reported to the MHRA.

There are some instances where it is important that all suspected ADRs are reported. These are as follows.

Black triangle drugs

Products that are first marketed are intensively monitored in order to confirm the risk/benefit profile of the product and are labelled with an inverted black triangle. Healthcare professionals are encouraged to report all suspected ADRs that occur as a result of the use of all black triangle drugs regardless of the seriousness of the reaction. Newly marketed products are usually intensively monitored for a minimum of 2 years; the black triangle is not necessarily removed after this time.

Any medication can be assigned a black triangle if it is considered that it needs to be intensively monitored. For example, black triangle status may be given to an established product if it is granted a new indication or route of administration, if it is marketed as a new combination with another established active ingredient, or if it is targeted towards a new patient population. If a product is a black triangle medicine this will be indicated in the BNF, the NPF, MIMS, and in the ABPI Compendium of Data Sheets and Summaries of Product Characteristics. Advertising material and patient information leaflets (PILs) should also include this information. A full list of all black triangle products and further information about the black triangle scheme can be found on the MHRA website at www.mhra.gov.uk.

Serious reactions

All serious suspected reactions must be reported regardless of whether or not a medicine is a black triangle drug or vaccine. The adverse effects of an established drug may be well known, but if a serious reaction occurs it should always be reported so that rare or delayed effects can be identified, more detailed advice can be given on potential side effects and comprehensive information can be used to compare the relative safety of medicines in the same therapeutic class. Reactions that are considered serious include those that:

- are fatal;
- are life threatening;
- are disabling or incapacitating;
- result in or prolong hospitalisation;
- result in congenital abnormalities;
- are medically significant.

For example, a review of cases reported via the Yellow Card Scheme led to the introduction of a warning on all aspirin products in October 2003 to highlight the risk of Reye's syndrome, which is associated with aspirin use in those aged below 16 years. Another example was the identification of a drug interaction that led to changes in international normalised ratio (INR) values following the concomitant administration of warfarin therapy with cranberry juice.

ADRs in children

The MHRA asks that all suspected ADRs occurring in children under the age of 18 years should be reported regardless of whether the medication is licensed for use in children. Children are often not exposed to medications during clinical trials and many medications are used in children even if they are not licensed for this purpose. This means that monitoring of drug safety is particularly important for this age group. In 2005 the first *BNF for Children* (BNFC) was launched, which gives 'practical information to help healthcare professionals who prescribe, monitor, supply, and administer medicines for childhood disorders'. This is a vital resource that can improve prescribing to children, and as with the BNF, the BNFC contains useful information that can help with the identification of ADRs. The BNFC clearly indicates whether or not a medication has a black triangle classification and also contains a few pre-paid Paper Yellow Cards, which can be used to report suspected ADRs.

CONCLUSION

This chapter has provided an overview to safety in medicines management.

COSHH and UICPs have been discussed. The principles of waste disposal and safe handling of medicines have been described. The procedure for reporting an ADR has been discussed.

REFERENCES

British Medical Association Board of Science (2006) *Reporting Adverse Drug Reactions. A Guide for Healthcare Professionals.* BMA, London. Available at www.bma.org.uk/images/ADRFinal_tcm41-20713.pdf.

Centers for Disease Control (1987) Recommendations for the prevention of HIV transmission in health care settings. *MMWR* **36**: 2S. Available at www.edc.gov/mmwr/preview/mmwrhtm/00023587.htm.

Centers for Disease Control (1999) NIOSH alert preventing needlestick injuries in healthcare settings. No. 2000-108. Available at www.cdc.gov/niosh/docs/2000-108/.

Department of Health (1998) *Guidance for Clinical Health Care Workers: Protection Against Infection with Blood-borne Viruses.* Recommendations of the Expert Advisory Group on AIDS and the Advisory Group on AIDS and the Advisory Group on Hepatitis. HMSO, London.

Department of Health (2006a) *Code of Practice for the Prevention and Control of Health Care Associated Infections.* HMS Crown Printing, London.

Department of Health (2006b) *Health Technical Memorandum 07–01: Safe Management of Healthcare Waste.* The Stationery Office, Norwich. Available at www.dh.gov.uk/en/Publicationsandstatistics/Publications/PublicationsPolicyAndGuidance/DH_063274.

Health and Safety Executive (2009) Working with substances hazardous to health. What you need to know about COSHH. Health and Safety Executive (HSE) INDG136 (rev4). Available at www.hse.gov.uk/pubns/indg136.pdf.

Health Protection Agency (2008) *Eye of the Needle. United Kingdom Surveillance of Significant Occupational Exposures to Bloodborne Viruses in Healthcare Workers.* Health Protection Agency, London. Available at www.hpa.org.uk/web/HPAwebFile/HPAweb_C/1227688128096.

National Institute for Clinical Excellence (NICE) (2003) Clinical Guideline 2. Infection Control: Prevention of healthcare-associated infection in primary and community care. NICE, London. Available at www.nice.org.uk/nicemedia/pdf/CG2fullguidelineinfectioncontrol.pdf.

National Patient Safety Alert (NPSA) (2004) Clean hands help to save lives. NPSA Patient Safety Alert 2 September 2004 superseded by an updated version on 2 September 2008. Available at www.nris.npsa.nhs.uk/resources/?entryid45=59848.

Royal Pharmaceutical Society of Great Britain (2005) *The Safe and Secure Handling of Medicines: A Team Approach.* A revision of the Duthie Report (1988) led by the Hospital Pharmacists' Group of the Royal Pharmaceutical Society. RPSGB, London. Available at www.rpsgb.org.uk/pdfs/safsechandmeds.pdf.

World Health Organization (WHO) (2009) WHO guidelines on hand hygiene in healthcare. WHO, Geneva. Available at whqlibdoc.who.int/publications/2009/9789241597906_eng.pdf.

FURTHER READING

Healthcare Professional Reporting of Adverse Drug Reactions: Frequently Asked Questions. MHRA, 22 October 2009. Available at www. mhra.gov.uk/Safetyinformation/Reportingsafetyproblems/ Medicines/Reportingsuspectedadversedrugreactions/ Healthcareprofessionalreporting/Frequentlyaskedquestions/ index.htm.

Royal Marsden Hospital (2008) *The Royal Marsden Hospital Manual of Clinical Nursing Procedures*, 7th edn. Wiley-Blackwell, Oxford.

Standard principles: personal protective equipment and the safe use and disposal of sharps. *Nursing Times.net*, 20 November 2007. Available at www.nursingtimes.net/nursing-practice-clinical-research/standard-principles-personal-protective-equipment-and-the-safe-use-and-disposal-of-sharps/291502.article.

4 Prescription of Medicines

Elizabeth Payne

INTRODUCTION

Prescribing has been the sole domain until the last decade of the medical/dental prescriber. However, this situation has changed to allow other healthcare professionals, particularly nurses, to take on this responsibility. This chapter will explore the elements of a prescription, particularly focusing on good practice when undertaking prescribing, the documentation used for prescribing and finally the methods whereby nurses may prescribe or supply and administer medicines without a prescription by a medical/dental prescriber.

The aim of this chapter is to provide an overview of the prescription of medicines.

LEARNING OUTCOMES

At the end of this chapter, the reader will be able to:

❑ Describe the essential elements of a prescription.
❑ Discuss the principles of safe prescribing.
❑ Discuss the use of prescription forms and prescription charts.
❑ Outline patient group directions (PGDs).
❑ Briefly discuss nurse prescribing.

ESSENTIAL ELEMENTS OF A PRESCRIPTION

One of the primary communication links between the prescriber, nurse, pharmacist and patient is complete, safe and accurate prescription writing. Completion of all 'essential elements' of a prescription ensures that it is accurately interpreted and not subject to alteration; this helps to ensure continuity of care. A prescription should be written legibly in ink or otherwise so as to be indelible.

The 'essential elements' of a prescription are described below [British National Formulary (BNF), 2009]:

- Patient name, hospital/NHS number, address, age (if child), date of birth and weight (if child)
  In secondary care, some of this information may be transmitted to the prescription by using the patient's addressograph label, although this is not ideal since the label can come off the prescription, hence patient details should be written clearly and unambiguously with black ballpoint in block capitals. The hospital number is essential to ensure that the intended patient receives the correct medication. It is not always necessary to provide the NHS number, age or weight. However, it is a legal requirement to state the age for children under 12 years in the case of prescription-only medicines. Furthermore, the patient's weight and height may be needed to calculate safe doses for many drugs with narrow therapeutic indices.
- Name, strength and dose of drug
  The internationally approved name (rINN), formulation (m/r tablets/capsules, transdermal patch, ear drops, etc.) and strength of the drug(s) should be written clearly, i.e. printed, if handwritten. Where different formulations and/or strengths of a preparation are available, it is important that details are correctly stated on the prescription, for example phenytoin suspension 30 mg/5 ml or 90 mg/5 ml. If an insulin or inhaler preparation is prescribed, it is important to state the device required to ensure that the patient receives the correct product.

  In secondary care, drugs have always been prescribed by the generic name, not by the proprietary or brand name, unless there is bio-inequivalence between brands (for example lithium, phenytoin, theophylline and carbamazepine, which are drugs with narrow therapeutic indices), potential for confusion (for example oral sustained-release opiates should be prescribed by brand name to reduce the risk of dispensing and administration errors) or a combination drug with no generic name (for example Tramacet®). This provides clarity regarding the drug required and ensures that the most cost-effective version of the drug can be supplied. This is not necessarily the case in primary care, where the prescriber may choose to prescribe a branded product if so wished.

  Abbreviations such as HCT, AZT, ISMN and T3 are not acceptable medical abbreviations, may be misinterpreted and may cause drug errors. A decimal point should not be used in doses unless unavoidable, for example 500 mg not 0.5 g, 100 micrograms not 0.1 mg. Where decimals are unavoidable a zero should be written in front of the decimal point where there is no other figure, for example 0.5 ml not .5 ml. Microgram and nanogram units should not be abbreviated but should always be written in full. For liquid preparations the dose should be written in milligrams; the only exceptions when millilitres may be used are if the product is a combination product such as Peptac® suspension or if the strength is not expressed in weight such as Adrenaline 1 in 1000. Numbers or figures, for example 1 or 'one', should be used to denote use of a sachet or enema.

- Quantity to be dispensed

  The quantity of drug to be dispensed should be given by indicating either the number of days of treatment required in the box provided on NHS forms or total quantity; this is necessary for primary care prescriptions and outpatient and discharge prescriptions in secondary care. The quantities of regular repeat prescriptions are generally limited to a maximum 28-day supply, with continuing supplies to be prescribed as refills. In order to minimise patient delays, the pharmacist is authorised to round the quantity dispensed to the nearest available pre-package quantity (usually a 1-month supply) only for prescriptions with refills authorised. In the case of controlled drugs (CDs), the total quantity should be written in words and figures, or the number of dosage units in words and figures, to prevent alteration of the prescription.

- Drug directions

  Clear and concise directions will assist patients in the appropriate use of the medication. *'Take as directed' should be avoided.* Patients may forget or confuse verbal directions or lose a separate note. Furthermore, directions on prescriptions should be written in complete English without abbreviation; it is recognised that some Latin abbreviations are used (see back cover of the *British National Formulary* (BNF)) such as OD for once a day, BD for twice a day, TDS for three times a day and QDS for four times a day. In the case of preparations to be taken 'as required', a *minimum dose interval* should be specified.

- Signature, printed name and date of prescription
  In addition to signing the prescription, it is good practice for the prescriber to print their name legibly next to their signature along with their registration number assigned by their regulatory authority.

  This will facilitate communications with healthcare professionals who have a need to accurately identify the prescriber, and it will also decrease the possibility of forgery. If the prescriber's signature is illegible and the identity of the prescriber is unknown, the prescription cannot be filled until the prescriber has been identified. This will result in delays to patients. To prevent illegal drug diversion, supplies of prescription blanks may not be signed by the prescriber in advance of use. A prescription must only be signed by the prescriber at the time it is written for a specific patient.
- Address of prescriber
  This is usually only required for primary care prescriptions or prescriptions issued from hospital for dispensing in primary care.

PRINCIPLES OF SAFE PRESCRIBING

Inadequate knowledge of patients and their clinical condition, inadequate knowledge of the drug, calculation errors, illegible handwriting, drug name confusion and poor history taking are among some of the reasons why prescribing errors occur. Prescribing error is potentially the most serious of all types of medication error as, unless detected, it may be repeated systematically for a prolonged period.

The Department of Health [Department of Health (DH), 2004] has published a document called *Building a Safer NHS for Patients: Improving Medication Safety*, which made the following recommendations for safe prescribing:

- Prescribers should be trained and assessed as competent before being required to prescribe, particularly in the case of anticoagulants and cytotoxic drugs. It is important that prescribers are familiar with what a legal prescription should document and feel confident with the medicines they commonly prescribe; the medicolegal responsibility for the prescription lies with the prescriber.

- The patient's medical record should always be checked before a new prescription is written so that the prescriber has adequate knowledge of the patient/client's health and medical needs. A new medicine should never be prescribed without a treatment plan wherein its effectiveness or otherwise is monitored.

- All paperwork used for prescribing medicines should include a section for allergy documentation and, if a new allergy is identified, the allergy record should be updated.

- Prescriptions should always carry patient directions and never be issued with the instruction 'as directed'. BNF guidance should be followed when writing prescriptions, and the completed prescription should be re-read to ensure that it is correct.

- All prescriptions for children should include the child's age and, where the dose is weight dependent, the child's weight and the intended dose in mg/kg.

- Particular attention should be paid to checking the accuracy of complex dose calculations. With respect to cytotoxic drugs, there should be a single method used by all staff for determining and checking body surface area within the organisation, and the patient's chemotherapy protocol should always be accessible by all staff involved in the patient's care.

- The treatment plan, including how the response to drug therapy is to be monitored and any subsequent changes to drug therapy, should be clearly documented in the patient's clinical notes.

- Where possible the aims and side effects of drug treatment should be discussed with the patient or their representative, as well as with other healthcare professionals involved in the patient's/client's care.

- Prescribers should have access to a pharmacist who is able to provide advice on the drug treatment plan. A guiding principle of professional bodies, such as the Nursing & Midwifery Council (NMC) or General Medical Council, is that prescribers should work within the limits of their competence.

- Prescribers should follow local and national prescribing standards, such as the British Society of Haematology guidelines, when prescribing anticoagulants.

- Where available, electronic prescribing systems should always be used for a number of reasons: all prescriptions include the drug name, dose, route and frequency (system prompts prescriber for these data elements); prescriptions are legible and the prescriber is always identifiable; information about the patient is available to the prescriber at the time of prescribing; information about the drug is available to the prescriber at the time of prescribing; prescribers are alerted to anomalous dose and frequency selection; prescriptions are checked for allergies, drug–drug interactions, drug–laboratory interactions, contraindications or cautions in the patient, and the prescriber is alerted; all relevant data about the patient and their drug regimen are available centrally; adverse effects can be documented and reported; audit and pharmacovigilance are facilitated; adverse drug events may be detected by capturing the use of antidotes such as vitamin K (warfarin overdose) or glucagon (insulin overdose), allowing a review of the events that led to their use; and relevant prescribing guidelines can be built into the prescribing system, helping to achieve optimal treatment.
- Actual and potential prescribing errors should be recorded and reviewed regularly to raise awareness of risk, and all serious prescribing errors and 'near misses' should be reported to the National Patient Safety Agency.

PRESCRIPTION FORMS

A number of different types of documentation are used for prescribing medicines, the most common being the prescription forms used in primary care, FP10NC (an example of an FP10NC may be found in the prescription writing section of the BNF), and a similar type used in hospital, FP10HNC, which may be dispensed by a community pharmacy as well as a hospital pharmacy (see form types below). In addition to the latter, hospital clinics may have their own in-house version of the FP10HNC, printed on a different background colour, which can only be dispensed by a hospital pharmacy. These forms are reserved mainly for ambulatory patients, unlike prescription charts used for in-patients admitted to an NHS Trust (Table 4.1).

Table 4.1 Prescription form versions and their purpose

Prescription form type	Colour	Purpose
FP10NC	Green	Hand-written prescription: prescriber details, address, etc. printed by manufacturer For use by GPs and hospitals
FP10SS	Green	Computer single-sheet prescription: prescription and prescriber name, address, etc. printed by computer prescribing system For use by GPs (and hospital/supplementary prescribers using accredited systems)
FP10MDA	Blue	Drug misuse instalment prescription: can be either pre-printed with prescriber name, address, etc. printed by manufacturer or 'occasional use' form for GPs, hospitals and supplementary prescribers or single-sheet blank forms with prescriber name, address, etc. printed by prescriber's computer prescribing system For use by GPs, hospitals and supplementary prescribers
FP10P	Lilac	Hand-written prescription pad: prescriber name, address, etc. and type of prescriber, e.g. 'Nurse Independent/ Supplementary Prescriber' printed by manufacturer For use by nurse, supplementary/additional prescribers and out-of-hours centres
FP10D	Yellow	Community dentist prescription
FP10PCDSS	Pink	Private controlled drug single-sheet prescription For use when prescribing controlled drugs in a private environment only
FP10PCDNC	Pink	Private controlled drug hand-written prescription For use when prescribing controlled drugs in a private environment only

Prescription forms are an important financial asset for the NHS, and theft and misuse can represent a huge financial loss. Stolen prescription forms, forgeries and medicines that are fraudulently obtained from a forgery are likely to be sold for substantial financial gains. Furthermore, these forms can be used to obtain medicines illegally, often CDs, for misuse. Medicines obtained in this way are often used for unsupervised treatment of an illness or health condition, to feed an addiction or for their performance-enhancing qualities. Without medical supervision or advice on possible adverse effects or contraindications to existing medical conditions, the consumers of these medicines put their health at significant risk and may even require urgent medical intervention. Prescription form theft and misuse can also contribute to violence.

Ensuring the security of prescription forms is a key area of action for the NHS Security Management Service (2008) (NHS SMS), which has, therefore, issued guidance entitled *Security of Prescription Forms Guidance-updated July 2008* to provide NHS health bodies in England with a framework for the development of policies, procedures and systems to ensure the security of prescription forms against theft and abuse.

Prescription forms normally change once a year. To keep forgery to a minimum, the guidance recommends that the latest version should be used. To help prescribers identify which version of prescriptions they should be using, all prescription forms have an identifier that includes the type of form, e.g. FP10HNC, and a date code, e.g. 0406. The form identifier is printed vertically in the Pricing Office box, e.g. FP10HNC0406 for FP10s, and underneath the prescriber's name and address box for instalment prescriptions. Details of all up-to-date prescription forms can be found on the NHS Business Services Authority website: www.nhsbsa.nhs.uk/PrescriptionServices/Documents/PrescriptionServices/Current_and_Out_of_Date_Rx_Form_Published_0709.pdf.

In addition to the prescription form identifier, each form also has a serial number that is positioned at the bottom of the form. The first 10 numbers are the serial number (these numbers run in sequence); the last (the 11th) character is a check digit and does not run in sequence. The serial number enables losses or thefts to be detected if the form(s) come into the prescription dispensing and processing systems.

The forms have a coloured background to make photocopying more difficult and contain chemical anti-tampering devices within both ink and paper to make unauthorised alterations (forgeries) detectable.

Personalisation on forms for handwritten use, e.g. FP10HNC, includes the Trust details, prescriber name, address telephone number and a prescriber/cost code number.

All prescription forms printed since April 1998 have a UV light-sensitive message. The UV message is included to aid detection of counterfeit forms. It is good practice for the prescriber to keep a record of the serial numbers of prescriptions issued to him/her, particularly the first and last serial numbers of the pads or computer forms. Recording the number of the first remaining prescription form of an in-use pad/box at the end of the working day is also recommended. These steps help to identify any prescriptions that are either lost or stolen overnight.

Blank prescription forms should not be pre-signed, to reduce the risk of misuse should they fall into the wrong hands. In addition, prescription forms should only be produced when needed and never left unattended. Prescription forms should not be left on a desk but placed in a drawer (which should be locked when the room is left unattended).

All unused forms should be returned to stock at the end of the session or day. Prescriptions are less likely to be stolen from (locked) secure stationery cupboards than from desks, bags or cars.

PRESCRIPTION CHARTS
Where a patient has been admitted to a residential or nursing home or secondary care facility, another form may be used for prescribing the patient's medication, such as a prescription chart. The purpose of a prescription chart is to provide a permanent record of the patient's medication and to direct and record the supply and administration of medicines.

There are many variations of prescription chart in use in the NHS, but most contain the following sections (Maxwell, 2007a, 2007b):

- *Basic patient information*, which identifies the prescription with the correct patient. This includes the patient's/client's name, date of birth, hospital unit number, ward address and consultant name and may include the patient/client's weight and height.
- *Previous adverse drug reactions/allergies* for communicating important patient/client safety information based on a careful medication history or the medical record: If a patient/client does not have any allergies, this should be recorded as no known drug allergies (NKDA); if a patient/client does have an allergy or a previous adverse drug reaction, as much information as possible regarding the type of allergy/adverse drug reaction should be documented on the chart. Medication may not be administered if this section is not completed by the prescriber.
- *Other medicines charts*: This section should be used to record any other medication charts in use, such as those used for anticoagulants, insulin and oxygen. As a general rule, it is good practice to record medicines prescribed on supplementary charts on the main chart, with a reference to the supplementary chart on the prescription. It is good practice to record multiple prescription charts as 1 of 2, 2 of 2.
- *Once-only medications*: This section is used for prescribing medicines to be used infrequently such as single-dose prophylactic antibiotics and other pre-operative medication.
- *Regular medications*: This section is for prescribing medicines to be taken for a number of days or continuously, such as a course of antibiotics, antihypertensive drugs, anti-Parkinsonian drugs, etc. Some NHS Trusts have separated antibiotics from regular medications and introduce an automatic stop for the former, usually after three days, unless the prescriber signs to authorise continuation. Each medicine should have the original start date charted, i.e. date of prescribing when patient/client was in hospital.

Besides the dose and frequency, the route of administration must be specified in the appropriate section; widely accepted abbreviations for route of administration are IV (intravenous), IM (intramuscular), SC (subcutaneous), SL (sublingual), PR (per rectum), PV (per vagina) and NG (nasogastric). 'Oral' and 'intrathecal' should never be abbreviated. Care should be taken in specifying 'right' or 'left' for eyedrops and eardops. Space is provided for each medication for notes on important administration advice such as whether a medicine should be taken with/after food or on an empty stomach.

If a course of treatment is for a known time period, subsequent days when the medicine is not required should be crossed off. If a medicine is not to be given every day, as in the case of weekly methotrexate or alendronic acid, the days when the medicine is not required should be crossed out. Discontinuation of an individual prescription should be done carefully with a vertical line at the point of discontinuation, horizontal lines through the remaining days on the prescription chart and diagonal lines through the prescription details and administration boxes; this action should be signed and dated by the prescriber. It is good practice to write a supplementary note to inform colleagues about the discontinuation.

- *As-required medications*: This section is for prescribing symptomatic relief, usually to be administered at the discretion of nursing staff, e.g. anti-emetics and analgesics. Prescribers should always note the indication, frequency, minimal time interval between doses and maximum dose in any 24-hour period.

NURSE PRESCRIBING

Nurse independent/supplementary prescribing emerged as a result of a drive to make better use of nurses' skills in delivering front-line care and to make it easier for patients to get access to medicines.

From November 2002, nurses were granted supplementary prescribing rights; this allowed nurse supplementary prescribers to prescribe for a full range of medical conditions under the terms of a clinical management plan agreed with a medical/dental prescriber and with the consent of the patient/client.

From 1 May 2006 changes to legislation allowed nurse independent prescribers (formerly extended formulary nurse prescribers) to prescribe any *licensed* medicine in the BNF (see part XVIIB(ii) of the drug tariff) for any medical condition that a nurse prescriber is competent to treat. This is ideal where the nurse prescriber works remotely from a medical/dental prescriber.

Furthermore, changes to the Misuse of Drug Regulations with the agreement of the Home Office's Advisory Council on the Misuse of Drugs enabled nurse independent prescribing of 13 CDs, but only for specific conditions, such as diamorphine and morphine for palliative care and post-operative pain relief. A list of these CDs and medical conditions is contained in the drug tariff (see part XVIIbii) and also in the BNF. For further information visit www.nhsbsa.nhs.uk/PrescriptionServices/924.aspx and www.bnf.org.uk.

All first-level registered nurses, registered midwives and registered specialist community public health nurses may be trained to be nurse independent/supplementary prescribers. However, the DH Guide to Implementation and the NMC Standards of Proficiency for nurse and midwife prescribers state that nurses put forward for prescribing training must have at least 3 years of post-registration experience.

Higher education institutions (HEIs) provide a specific programme of preparation and training for independent prescribing, which are approved by the Nursing & Midwifery Council and the Royal Pharmaceutical Society of Great Britain. Nurses who successfully complete the programme must register their prescribing qualification with the Nursing & Midwifery Council before they can start prescribing. For further information, visit www.nmc-uk.org.

Prescribing training courses are centrally funded through Strategic Health Authority Workforce Directorates. The training course is spread over a period of 6 months and consists of at least 26 days training and 12 days learning in practice. A designated medical practitioner must supervise the student and provide support, and there are elements of self-directed learning. A buddying system using another qualified independent prescriber may also be very beneficial. Previous learning can be taken into account through the accreditation of prior learning, at the discretion of the HEI, and some elements of the course can be delivered through distance learning. All participants must pass the end of course assessments.

More detailed information about nurse prescribers is given in Chapter 14.

PATIENT GROUP DIRECTIONS

The use of group protocols, which allowed non-prescribers to supply or administer medicines, used to be commonplace in the NHS. The legal framework that allowed such supply to continue, if it was consistent with the legal framework, using patient group directions (PGDs), was set up and put in place in August 2000.

A PGD is a written instruction for the supply or administration of a *licensed* medicine (or medicines), without a prescription, in an identified clinical situation, where the patient/client may not be individually identified before presenting for treatment. This should not be interpreted as indicating that the patient *must* not be identified; patients may or may not be identified, depending on the circumstances.

The majority of clinical care should be provided on an individual, patient-specific basis. A PGD should only be developed where it will:

- improve access to treatment;
- offer an advantage to patient care without compromising patient safety, i.e. where there are 'high-volume' groups of patients who present for treatment, such as people needing vaccines or 'routine' treatments such as eyedrops before clinical examination;
- reduce patient waiting times;
- ensure the appropriate use and extension of the skills used by the various healthcare professionals detailed in the legislation.

PGDs are not a form of prescribing and are not suitable where a range of different medicines needs to be given to the patient at the same time; PGDs are not meant to be a long-term means of managing a patient's clinical condition.

A PGD should be drawn up by a multidisciplinary group involving a medical/dental prescriber, pharmacist and other healthcare professionals from the group to whom the PGD will apply (for example, nurse if the PGD will apply to a nurse). Each PGD must be signed by the medical/dental prescriber and pharmacist involved in developing the PGD, and approved by the organisation in which it is to be used, typically a primary care trust (PCT) or NHS Trust. This process may be assigned to the local Drug and Therapeutics Committee. Electronic signatures can be used to sign off a PGD as long as the electronic signature is linked uniquely to an individual and under their sole control.

The organisations that are eligible to sell, supply and administer medicines under PGDs are:

- special health authorities;
- NHS Trusts and PCTs;
- a doctor's or dentist's practice, in the provision of NHS services;
- a non-NHS organisation providing treatment under an arrangement made with an NHS Trust or PCT (e.g. a walk-in centre or family planning clinic);
- services funded by the NHS but provided by the private, voluntary or charitable sector;
- independent hospitals, agencies and clinics registered under the Care Standards Act 2000;
- healthcare services provided by the prison service;
- healthcare services provided by the police force;
- healthcare services provided by the medical service for the armed forces.

PGDs can only be used by the following registered healthcare professionals, acting as named individuals: nurses, midwives, health visitors, paramedics, optometrists, chiropodists and podiatrists, radiographers, orthoptists, physiotherapists, pharmacists, dieticians, occupational therapists, prosthetists and orthotists, and speech and language therapists.

Each PGD has a list of individuals named as competent to supply/administer under the direction; this generally takes the form of signatures and names (on a list of individual forms) that are attached to the PGD itself or held by the service or organisation. There are no specific national training programmes for PGDs; it is the responsibility of individual organisations to ensure that professionals supplying/administering medicines under a PGD are competent to do so, hence a senior person in each profession locally should be designated with the responsibility to ensure that registered and trained professionals operate within their own expertise and competence when using PGDs and understand that they cannot delegate the supply or administration of medicines to another nurse or healthcare professional. The National Prescribing Centre (NPC, 2009) has developed an outline competency framework for local use. It should be noted that not every practitioner is expected to use PGDs. Patient and service need should be considered when deciding who needs to use them.

Legislation (see also HSC 2000/26: www.dh.gov.uk) requires that each PGD must contain the following information:

- the name of the business to which the direction applies;
- the date the direction comes into force and the date it expires;
- a description of the medicine(s) to which the direction applies;
- the class of health professional who may supply or administer the medicine;
- the signature of a doctor or dentist, as appropriate, and a pharmacist;
- the signature of an appropriate health organisation;
- the clinical condition or situation to which the direction applies;
- a description of those patients excluded from treatment under the direction;
- a description of the circumstances in which further advice should be sought from a doctor (or dentist, as appropriate) and arrangements for referral;
- details of appropriate dosage and maximum total dosage, quantity, pharmaceutical form and strength, route and frequency of administration, and minimum and maximum period over which the medicine should be administered. The medical prescriber/pharmacist signing the PGD must be satisfied that the dose range is clinically appropriate and within the terms of the medicine's marketing authorisation. The clinical criteria for selecting a dose within the range must be specified;
- relevant warnings, including potential adverse reactions;
- details of any necessary follow-up action and the circumstances;
- a statement of the records to be kept for audit purposes.

National template PGDs are accessible via the National Electronic Library for Health website at www.portal.nelm.nhs. uk/PGD/default.aspx. Legally a PGD should be formally reviewed and re-authorised every 2 years and the review date should be included in the PGD.

Black triangle drugs (i.e. those recently licensed and subject to special reporting arrangements for adverse reactions) and medicines used outside the terms of the summary of product characteristics (e.g. as used in some areas of specialist paediatric care) may be included in PGDs, provided such use is exceptional, justified by current best clinical practice and that a direction clearly describes the status of the product. Where the medicine is for children, particular attention will be needed to specify any restrictions on the age, size and maturity of the child. Each PGD should clearly state when the product is being used outside the terms of the SPC, and the documentation should include the reasons why, exceptionally, such use is necessary.

Nurses can *supply* and *administer* some CDs under the terms of a PGD. PGDs can be used for the supply and administration of Schedule 4 Part 1 CDs (mostly benzodiazepines) but not in a parenteral form for the treatment of addiction and schedule 5 CDs (low-strength opiates such as codeine), with the exception of anabolic steroids. Note that Midazolam has been re-scheduled from schedule 4 to schedule 3, but its use will continue to be allowed under a PGD. In addition, but limited to nurses in accident and emergency departments and in coronary care units in hospitals, diamorphine can be supplied/administered for the treatment of cardiac pain.

Caution is required in the development of PGDs related to antimicrobial agents. A local microbiologist should be involved in drawing up these PGDs to ensure that their development will not jeopardise strategies to combat resistance to antimicrobial agents.

The administration of radiopharmaceuticals is regulated by the Medicines (Administration of Radioactive Substances) Regulations 1978 and should not be included in PGDs.

Neither unlicensed medicines nor appliances or dressings can be supplied or administered under a PGD, as PGDs only apply to licensed medicines. Dressings and appliances can be provided using a protocol or guidelines, or they can be prescribed by an appropriately qualified independent nurse prescriber.

Medicines for PGD use should be available as pre-packs already labelled with the relevant details by pharmacy staff [Royal Pharmaceutical Society of Great Britain (RPSGB), 2008]. The professional supplying the medicine can then add the patient's/client's name and date. The patient information leaflet (PIL) must be included with the supply. If the PIL is not available in the pack, it can be found on the electronic medicines compendium and printed to be included in the supply of the medicine.

More detailed information about PGDs is available from the National Prescribing Centre's publication on PGDs (2009), available at www.npc.co.uk/prescribers/resources/patient_group_directions.pdf, and in *Health Service Circular (HSC) 2000/026 Patient Group Directions [England only]*, available at www.dh.gov.uk/publications (DH, 2000).

CONCLUSION

This chapter has provided an overview to the prescription of medicines. The essential elements of a prescription have been described. The principles of safe prescribing, together with the use of prescription forms and prescription charts, have been discussed. PGDs have been discussed and a brief introduction to nurse prescribing has been provided.

REFERENCES

British National Formulary (BNF) (2009) *Prescription Writing*. BMJ Publishing Group Ltd, London, and RPS Publishing, London.

Department of Health (DH) (2000) *Patient Group Directions (England only) HSC 2000/026*. Department of Health, London. Available at www.dh.gov.uk/publications [accessed on 4 November 2009].

Department of Health (DH) (2004) *Building a Safer NHS for Patients. Improving Medication Safety*. Available at www.dh.gov.uk/en/Publicationsandstatistics/Publications/PublicationsPolicyAndGuidance/DH_4071443 [accessed on 4 November 2009].

Maxwell SRJ, Wilkinson K (2007a) The medic's guide to prescribing: safe and effective prescribing. *StudentBMJ* **15**: 169–212.

Maxwell SRJ, Wilkinson K (2007b) Writing safe and effective prescriptions in a hospital kardex. *J R Coll Physicians Edinb* **37**: 348–351.

National Prescribing Centre (2009) *Patient Group Directions – a Practical Guide and Framework of Competencies for All Professionals Using Patient Group Directions.* National Prescribing Centre, Liverpool. Available at www.npc.co.uk/prescribers/resources/patient_group_directions.pdf

NHS Security Management Service (2008) *Security of Prescription Forms Guidance.* Available at www.dhsspsni.gov.uk/pas-security-prescription-forms-guidance-feb08.pdf [accessed in February 2008]

Royal Pharmaceutical Society of Great Britain (RPSGB) (2008) *Legal and Ethical Advisory Service Fact Sheet: Seven Patient Group Directions: a Resource Pack for Pharmacists.* Royal Pharmaceutical Society of Great Britain, London. Available at www.rpsgb.org.uk/pdfs/factsheet7.pdf

5 | Systems for Medicines Administration

Kate Roland and Ruth Endacott

INTRODUCTION

Systems for medicines administration may describe storage systems for medicines as well as the process by which medicines are administered.

The term 'medicine', when used in this chapter, refers to all prescribed or over-the-counter medication. It is a general term that includes tablets, capsules, liquids, inhalers, eye drops, creams, ointments, suppositories and patches.

All hospitals should have a medicines management policy relating to the safe storage, supply, handling and administration of medicines [Royal Pharmaceutical Society of Great Britain (RPSGB), 2005]. Legislation applies to the prescribing, supply, storage and administration of medicines. It is essential to be aware of and comply with this legislation [Nursing & Midwifery Council (NMC), 2008; RPSGB, 2009].

LEARNING OUTCOMES

At the end of this chapter, the reader will be able to:

❏ Describe hospital-based systems for medicines administration.
❏ Discuss the principles of self-administration.
❏ Describe community-based systems for medicines administration.

HOSPITAL-BASED SYSTEMS FOR MEDICINES ADMINISTRATION

Hospital-based systems for medicines administration can include the following:

• administration from stock cupboards;
• administration from drug trolleys;

- administration from bedside lockers;
- one-stop dispensing schemes;
- patient's own drugs (POD) schemes.

All medicines must be stored securely in a lockable cabinet or cupboard. This can be a ward stock cupboard, lockable drug trolley or bedside locker (RPSGB, 2005). Medicines used for administration may be ward stock, an inpatient non-stock supply, without directions for use, or a patient's own supply, which is labelled with the patient's name and clear directions for use.

Traditionally, medicines administered in hospital were ward stock drugs or inpatient supplies taken from stock cupboards or drug trolleys and given out to patients on a drug round (Commission for Healthcare Audit and Inspection, 2007). Many trusts now have bedside lockers for the storage of medicines. Administration of medicines from bedside lockers can make the process a more personal experience and give patients an opportunity to discuss, and ask questions about, their medicines (Commission for Healthcare Audit and Inspection, 2007). Bedside lockers also facilitate administration schemes such as one-stop dispensing, POD and self-medication (Commission for Healthcare Audit and Inspection, 2007).

One-stop dispensing and POD schemes have changed the way medication is administered in hospitals (Commission for Healthcare Audit and Inspection, 2007). One-stop dispensing schemes involve the use of the patient's own medicines whilst they are inpatients, those dispensed in the community or by the hospital pharmacy or both. The medicines must be labelled with full instructions for use and contain a patient information leaflet (NMC, 2008). Supplies are monitored and topped up when they run out or when new medicines are prescribed. Medicines supplied during admission are dispensed ready for discharge (NMC, 2008); one-stop dispensing is also known as dispensing for discharge. Some drugs are not suitable for supply under a one-stop dispensing scheme. This may be because the dose is highly variable or being titrated up or down, or because the drug will not be prescribed on discharge, for example analgesics, including controlled drugs, antibiotics and injectable (intravenous, intramuscular or subcutaneous) drugs.

POD schemes are part of the one-stop dispensing process. PODs are those that patients bring in from home; they may be prescribed, over-the-counter or alternative medicines. PODs must be assessed before use by pharmacy or nursing staff, according to local policy. The medicines must be suitable for use, e.g. in date, labelled correctly, in suitable packaging/container and labelled with the patient's name. All POD schemes will have assessment criteria, which much be adhered to.

Patients must give consent for their medication to be used during their inpatient stay. PODs are a patient's property and cannot be removed or destroyed without the patient's permission. Any PODs that are deemed unsuitable for use or that have been stopped during admission should ideally be disposed of. If the patient does not give permission, the PODs should be returned to the patient on discharge and the patient advised that these should be disposed of and why. PODs must only be given to the patient they belong to and never to other patients.

Controlled drugs should be stored in the ward controlled drug cupboard, according to Controlled Drugs Regulations (RPSGB, 2009) and appropriate records must be kept. Patients' own controlled drugs should also be stored in the ward controlled drugs cupboard and recorded in a separate section of the controlled drugs register, unless local policy allows otherwise.

One-stop dispensing and POD schemes facilitate faster discharge, assuming that a patient's condition is stable and frequent changes to medication are not needed. The use of individually dispensed medicines also reduces the risk of administration errors that may occur when medicines are administered from ward or inpatient stock (Commission for Healthcare Audit and Inspection, 2007). Use of PODs can also achieve cost savings for the Trust as less medication is wasted (Commission for Healthcare Audit and Inspection, 2007). PODs are also a valuable resource when reconciling a patient's medication history on admission [National Institute for Health and Clinical Excellence (NICE), 2007].

Electronic systems to support prescribing and administration

Electronic prescribing is a key feature of patient safety policy in a number of countries (Smith, 2004). Systems for electronic prescribing range from computerised order entry (Shulman *et al.*, 2005) to fully integrated prescribing, dispensing and administration systems (Barber *et al.*, 2007). Fully integrated systems comprise prescribing, dispensing, administering and reviewing (see Table 5.1).

Studies investigating the impact of electronic prescribing on error rates show variable findings (Han *et al.*, 2005; Nebeker *et al.*, 2005; Shulman *et al.*, 2005), suggesting that there are organisational factors to take into account when setting up electronic systems. Franklin and colleagues (2007) found that there were significant reductions in prescribing errors ($p < 0.001$) and major adverse events ($p = 0.005$) with improvement in the checking of patient identity ($p < 0.001$) when electronic prescribing was implemented as part of an integrated system, although there were also increases in time spent by pharmacists and medical staff on medication-related tasks (Franklin *et al.*, 2007). A further

Table 5.1 Components of a fully integrated electronic medicines management system

Component	Detail
Prescribing	Undertaken either at the bedside using a portable computer or at a central workstation
	Access to patient's entire medication history for current admission
Dispensing	Ward-based console for loading of drug trolley
	Nurses use touch screen to select drugs for loading into the drug trolley
Administration	Drugs administered to the patient from a drug trolley with electronically locked individual drawers for each patient
	Patient's bar-coded wristband read by scanner on the drugs trolley
	Correct scanning opens the drawer for that patient
Prescription review	Prescribing data reviewed by pharmacists at a workstation on the ward or at a console in the pharmacy department
	Pharmacists have 'read and write' access to the patient's medication prescription

Adapted from Barber *et al.* (2007).

study showed that electronic prescribing can decrease nurse time but increase medical time (Poissant *et al.*, 2005).

Electronic systems also require additional safeguards to avoid 'juxtaposition errors' (Ash *et al.*, 2004).These can occur when two medications are in close proximity on the prescribing screen. In the same way, some systems allow easy movement between records for different patients and require extra vigilance to avoid errors.

One advantage of electronic prescribing is the requirement to follow protocols, for example not allowing doctors to omit information when prescribing a medication, although additional errors may be introduced for medications with varying doses or times, such as sliding scale insulin or variable-dose heparin, that do not easily fit into the 'system' (Barber *et al.*, 2007).

PRINCIPLES OF SELF-MEDICATION

Self-medication schemes allow patients to administer their own medication whilst in hospital, under the supervision of nursing staff. Self-medication is also known as self-administration.

Self-administration of medicines has been advocated by various healthcare bodies, including the NMC (2008), Audit Commission (2001, 2002), Commission for Healthcare Audit and Inspection (2007) and the United Kingdom Hospital Pharmacists Group (2002). The National Service Framework for older people issued by the Department of Health (DH) recommends the use of self-administration schemes as a method of improving patient compliance and addressing any medication-related problems before discharge (DH, 2001).

Organisations must have a self-administration policy in place which covers the use of patients' own medicines and ensures that there is a safe and secure process for the storage, supply, handling and administration of these medicines (RPSGB, 2005). Self-medication requires the use of medication labelled with the patient's name and appropriate directions for use. Self-medication schemes usually run alongside a POD or one-stop dispensing scheme, as described above.

All medicines for patient self-medication must be stored securely in a locked cabinet or cupboard accessible to the patient (RPSGB, 2005). Many hospitals have lockable bedside lockers or cabinets in which medication can be stored. Depending on local policy, patients may be given a key to this locker to enable them to self-administer.

A patient must be assessed as being suitable to self-administer in hospital. Assessment may be carried out by nursing or pharmacy staff, according to local policy. Patients must give their consent for self-medication. If patients are not able to self-administer or do not wish to, nursing staff should administer their medication during their stay in hospital. Patients have the right to withdraw their consent at any time.

Self-administration is not suitable in the following situations:

- If the patient is confused or disorientated to time and/or place.
- If the patient has a history of drug or alcohol abuse or suicidal tendencies.
- If the patient is undergoing a test, procedure or operation that requires them to be sedated or have a general anaesthetic.
- Patients may not be allowed to self-administer controlled drugs, such as morphine. This will depend on local policy.
- If any alterations are made to a patient's medication or new medication is started, these drugs are usually given by nursing staff until the patient becomes familiar with them. Once the nurse and patient are happy, a patient may begin to self-administer these items.
- Some medication may not be suitable for self-administration, e.g. intravenous medication and controlled drugs.

Patients will vary in their abilities and needs with regard to their medication. Different levels of self-administration should be used to allow for this (see Table 5.2).

Self-medication schemes should be flexible and patients able to move between levels as appropriate during their hospital stay. Patients must be regularly reassessed to ensure that they are still able to self-administer.

As with all medicines administration, when supervising a patient self-medicating, it is essential that you understand what the medication is, why the patient is taking it and the dose they should be taking. Knowledge of a drug's potential side effects, cautions and contraindications is also vital. If you are at all unsure, seek clarification from the prescriber, pharmacist, doctor,

Table 5.2 Levels of medication self-administration

Level 0	Full nurse administration	All medicines are administered by nursing staff
Level 1	Full supervision	Nurses and/or other healthcare professionals teach the patient/carers what the purpose of the medication is and how to administer it The nurse may still administer the medication
Level 2	Close supervision	Patients request their medication from nursing staff at the appropriate times Patients are self-administering but checking medication with nurses
Level 3	Full self-administration	Patients are allowed to administer their medication themselves without any supervision Patients should be given responsibility for the key to their drug locker or cabinet

senior colleague or the current edition of the *British National Formulary* (BNF).

Self-medication has both advantages and disadvantages. These are described in Table 5.3.

Self-medication provides an opportunity to identify any problems patients might have with their medicines. These could include side effects, physical problems such as poor eyesight or poor dexterity, or poor memory. It is important to be aware of how these problems could be overcome. A pharmacist or pharmacy technician will be able to give advice regarding appropriate ways to help. Some of the potential solutions are discussed in more detail below.

COMMUNITY-BASED SYSTEMS FOR MEDICINES ADMINISTRATION

Community-based systems for medicines administration focus on supporting patients who have practical problems adhering to their medication. There is no single solution that applies to all patients. Support with adherence must be tailored to address an individual's specific needs at a specific time. These needs

Table 5.3 Advantages and disadvantages of medication self-administration

Advantages	Disadvantages
Allows patients to become familiar with their medication whilst in a safe environment	Not suitable for all patients
Allows identification of any problems patients have with their medication, e.g. side effects, problems with eyesight or memory, and difficulties opening packs or bottles	Patients may not want to self-medicate
Allows assessment of any potential support methods, e.g. reminder charts and monitored dosage systems	Not suitable for all types of medication, e.g. intravenous drugs, new medication if unfamiliar and controlled drugs (depending on local policy)
May increase patient concordance with the medication	May be potential safety issues, e.g. over- or under-dosing – accidental or intentional
May increase patients' understanding and knowledge of their medication	Medication must be managed across primary and secondary care interface to ensure that medication remains the same on discharge
May reduce medication errors	Self-medication schemes can be time-consuming to set up
Can improve patient comfort as they can administer their medication at times when they need it, e.g. analgesia, sleeping tablets and Parkinson's medication	
Allows patients to become involved in their care and make decisions about their treatment	
Demonstrates trust in the patient and promotes independence, which can have psychological benefits	
May save nursing time once patient is self-medicating, as fewer medicines need to be given by nursing staff	

may change over time, so support systems must be regularly reassessed to ensure that they are still appropriate. Adherence should be assessed every time a medicine is prescribed, dispensed or reviewed by any healthcare professional. Good communication between patient and healthcare professional is essential (NICE, 2009).

The NICE released guidance on medicines adherence in January 2009 (NICE, 2009). This guidance offers best practice advice on how to involve patients in decisions about their pre-scribed medicines and how to support adherence (NICE, 2009). NICE describes two categories of non-adherence to medication: intentional, where the patient chooses not to take medication as prescribed, and unintentional, where the patient wants to take the medication but is unable to due to practical problems.

Intentional non-adherence can be addressed by involving patients in decision making about their medication and making sure that they have sufficient, appropriate information to make these decisions (NICE, 2009). It is important to acknowledge that patients have the right to choose whether to take medication or not, as long as they have the capacity to make this decision. Patients must be provided with the necessary information to make an informed choice and be given the opportunity to become involved in decision making about their medicines (NICE, 2009).

Community-based systems for medicines administration tend to support patients who are unintentionally non-adherent. Unintentional non-adherence can be addressed by assessing the practical problems and intervening where appropriate. Evidence for practical intervention is inconclusive, therefore interventions should only be made if there is a specific need (Bhattacharya, 2005; NICE, 2009).

The Disability Discrimination Act requires pharmacists and prescribers to make 'reasonable' adjustments to support patients with long-term impairment to take their medication. These adjustments include provision of 'auxiliary aids' or interventions to assist with adherence. Auxiliary aids are considered to be anything that may assist patients to manage their medication. Pharmacies should make an assessment of a patient's needs and offer appropriate advice and support (Pharmaceutical Services Negotiating Committee, 2005).

Practical problems with medicines and some potential inter-ventions are described in Table 5.4.

Multicompartment compliance aids can be used to assist indi-viduals with memory problems or complex medication regimes.

Table 5.4 Practical problems and potential interventions for medicines administration

Practical problem	Potential intervention
Physical problems, e.g. poor dexterity, lack of strength to open packaging	Use of non-click-lock or easy-open lids for bottles
	Devices to help with the administration of eye drops or aerosol inhalers
	Devices to help remove tablets or capsules from foil or blister packs
	Devices to help squeeze creams and ointments from tubes
	Multi-compartment compliance aids
Visual impairment	Large print, coloured or Braille labels
	Audio versions of patient information leaflets
Poor memory	Medicines reminder charts
	Medicines administration charts or tick charts
	Alarm clocks to prompt administration
	Multi-compartment compliance aids
Communication problems, e.g. inability to read medicine labels or patient information leaflets due to reading or language difficulties	Audio versions of patient information leaflets
	Translations of patient information leaflet and administration instructions
Poor understanding of medicines	Appropriate patient information
	Medicines reminder chart
Unable to swallow solid-dose formulations	Liaise with pharmacy/prescriber to change formulation of medicines, e.g. liquids, patches
	Tablet cutters and crushers available if appropriate
	Note: Crushing of tablets/opening of capsules is unlicensed and may not be appropriate or safe – always seek advice from a pharmacist before advising a patient to do this
Unable to use devices, e.g. inhalers	Education
	Use of aids such as a Haleraid®
	Change to alternative inhaler device
Problems accessing medicines, e.g. needs help to order and collect medicines	Assistance with ordering of medicines
	Collection and delivery service for medicines

These compliance aids are also known as monitored dosage systems (MDS). There are a number of multicompartment compliance aids available. These aids usually contain a week's worth of medication in separate slots for times of day and days of the week.

Multicompartment compliance aids can be divided into two types: patient-filled compliance aids and pharmacy-dispensed compliance aids. The choice of aid used will depend on the individual's needs and abilities.

Patient-filled compliance aids are available to buy in pharmacies and other shops, in various shapes and sizes. These include Medidos® and Medimax® tablet dispensers, pill towers, and daily or weekly pill organisers. Compliance aids are available with built-in alarms to prompt administration. These aids must be filled by the patient or a friend, family member or carer. Patient-filled aids are not sealed and therefore can be altered after filling. This makes these systems more flexible if amendments to medication are needed. However, the potential for alteration raises a number of safety/clinical governance issues. For example, it is difficult to identify individual tablets and therefore monitor if the correct medicines have been taken. Also, alterations to the pack may not be immediately obvious. The person filling the compliance aid takes responsibility for filling it correctly according to the prescriber's instructions. There is the potential for error due to secondary dispensing from previously dispensed packs (Bhattacharya, 2005). Patients or carers may need support with this initially until they are confident to manage alone. Some patients or carers may not want to take on this responsibility; this is entirely their choice. In this situation, a pharmacy-filled device may be more appropriate. Filling of compliance aids by nurses is classed as dispensing by the NMC, and should only occur if the employer is aware and the practice is covered by a standard operating procedure (NMC, 2008). Nurses who fill compliance aids for patients are recommended to confirm that the medications have been packaged appropriately, to ensure that standards of medication labelling and conditions of the product licence are maintained.

Pharmacy-dispensed compliance aids, such as 'blister' or 'bubble' packs or NOMAD® trays, are only available from pharmacies. Medication is dispensed directly into these aids by the pharmacy, and they are sealed once filled. This makes amendment more difficult but makes the compliance aid safer as alterations are obvious. Some pharmacies will also fill unsealed Medidos® type containers.

Table 5.5 Advantages and disadvantages of using medicine compliance aids

Advantages	Disadvantages
Act as a memory aid	Error risk from secondary dispensing, e.g. if aids filled at home from original packs dispensed by community or hospital pharmacy
Visual prompt for patient or carers that patient has taken medication	Difficult to identify individual tablets, e.g. if omission required or the patient does not want to take a specific medication
Can help to manage complex medicine regimes, e.g. Parkinson's medication	Packaging is not child resistant
Minimise dose amount and timing errors	Risk of doses being lost or mixed up if unsealed pack is dropped or tampered with
Provide medicines storage that is easier for the patient to access, e.g. if patient has difficulty with medicine packaging due to poor dexterity	Requires weekly prescriptions – more expensive than monthly dispensing
Patient-filled aids may be useful for over-the-counter or alternative medicines that would not be put into pharmacy-dispensed compliance aids	Some pharmacies charge for supply of dispensed compliance aids
	Non-pharmacy-dispensed aids need to be filled weekly – requires someone to do this
	Filling of compliance aids is time-consuming
	Reduces flexibility in dosing as aids are filled weekly
	Only suitable for tablets and capsules that are to be swallowed whole
	Stability issues – long-term stability of medicines in pack unknown, not all medication is suitable to go into a compliance aid for stability reasons
	Limited space for each dose – may not fit all medicines in
	Patient must be able to understand how the aid is used
	If started in hospital, supply must be arranged to continue on discharge

Compliance aids such as these can be given to patients in hospital and on discharge. They are often used in conjunction with self-medication schemes. However, on discharge it is essential that arrangements are made for them to be filled or supplied in the community.

In some parts of the UK, pharmacy-dispensed compliance aids are required by care agencies in order for carers to prompt or administer a patient's medicines. Nursing homes often have a similar pharmacy-dispensed system for residents' medication.

Multicompartment compliance aids can be useful in managing medicines administration for some patients. However, they are not always the appropriate solution. Some of the advantages and disadvantages of the use of compliance aids are given in Table 5.5 (Bhattacharya, 2005).

CONCLUSION

There are a variety of systems for medicines administration in hospital and community settings. It is essential to be aware of the systems used in your organisation, and the policies and procedures that support them. No one system is suitable for everyone, so it is important to be aware of the uses and limitations of each to ensure that you are practicing appropriately.

REFERENCES

Ash JS, Berg M, Coiera E (2004) Some unintended consequences of information technology in health care: the nature of patient care information system-related errors. *J Am Med Inform Assoc* **11**: 104–112.

Audit Commission (2001) *A Spoonful of Sugar – Medicines Management in NHS Hospitals*. Audit Commission, London.

Audit Commission (2002) *Medicines Management – Review of National Findings*. Audit Commission, London.

Barber N, Cornford T, Klecun E (2007) Qualitative evaluation of an electronic prescribing and administration system. *Qual Saf Health Care* **16**: 271–278.

Bhattacharya D (2005) *Indications for Multi compartment Compliance Aids (MCA) Provision*. Available at www.pcc.nhs.uk/uploads/2005_Apr/Literature%20Review%20of%20Indications%20for%20monitored%20dosage%20system%20provision.doc [accessed on 19 July 2009].

Commission for Healthcare Audit and Inspection (2007) *The Best Medicine – The Management of Medicines in Acute and Specialist Trusts*. Commission for Healthcare Audit and Inspection, London.

Department of Health (DH) (2001) *Medicines & Older People – Implementing Medicines-Related Aspects of the NSF for Older People*. DH, London.

Franklin BD, O'Grady K, Donyai P, Jacklin A, Barber N (2007) The impact of a closed-loop electronic prescribing and administration system on prescribing errors, administration errors and staff time: a before-and-after study. *Qual Saf Health Care* **16**: 279–284.

Han YY, Carcillo JA, Venkataraman ST, *et al.* (2005) Unexpected increased mortality after implementation of a commercially sold computerized physician order system. *Pediatrics* **116**(6): 1506–1512.

Hospital Pharmacists Group (2002) One-stop dispensing, use of patients' own drugs and self-administration schemes. *Hosp Pharm* **9**(3): 81–86.

National Institute for Health and Clinical Excellence (NICE) (2007) *Technical Patient Safety Solutions for Medicines Reconciliation on Admission of Adults to Hospital*. National Institute for Health and Clinical Excellence, London.

National Institute for Health and Clinical Excellence (NICE) (2009) *Medicines Adherence – Involving Patients in Decisions About Prescribed Medicines and Supporting Adherence*. National Institute for Health and Clinical Excellence, London.

Nebeker JR, Hoffman JM, Weir CR, Bennett CL, Hurdle JF (2005) High rates of adverse drug events in a highly computerized hospital. *Arch Intern Med* **165**(10): 1111–1116.

Nursing & Midwifery Council (NMC) (2008) *Standards for Medicines Management*. NMC, London.

Pharmaceutical Services Negotiating Committee (2005) *PSNC Guidance for Pharmacy Contractors – Disability Discrimination Act 1995 – Support for People with Disabilities*. Available at www.psnc.org.uk/publications_detail.php/195/guidance_on_the_disability_discrimination_act_1995 [accessed on 19 July 2009].

Poissant L, Pereira J, Tamblyn R, *et al.* (2005) The impact of electronic health records on time efficiency of physicians and nurses. *J Med Inform Assoc* **12**: 505–516.

Royal Pharmaceutical Society of Great Britain (RPSGB) (2005) *The Safe and Secure Handling of Medicines: A Team Approach*. RPSGB, London.

Royal Pharmaceutical Society of Great Britain (RPSGB) (2009) *Medicines, Ethics and Practice: A Guide for Pharmacists and Pharmacy Technicians*. RPSGB, London.

Shulman R, Singer M, Goldstone J, *et al.* (2005) Medication errors: a prospective cohort study of hand-written and computerised physician order entry in the intensive care unit. *Crit Care* **9**: R516–R521.

Smith J (2004) *Building a Safer NHS for Patients: Improving Medication Safety*. Department of Health, London.

6 | Principles of Safe Administration of Medicines

Dan Higgins

INTRODUCTION

A medical prescription is one of the most common treatments in the NHS. GPs in England issue more than 660 million prescriptions every year; it is estimated that an additional 200 million prescriptions per year are generated in a hospital setting [Department of Health (DH), 2004]. Nurses are responsible for the majority of medication administration in the UK (Wright, 2009). This process involves considerable risk and as such nurses must endeavour to ensure that the whole process is undertaken with the highest regard for safety.

The process of medicines administration will always be accompanied by a degree of risk that can be attributed to errors in the prescribing, dispensing of and finally the administration of these medicines to the patient. The risks may be unpredictable, for example the patient may experience an adverse effect as a consequence of taking a particular medication. A patient may also experience side effects as a result of medicine administration; whilst not an adverse event, a side effect describes a response that is judged to be secondary to the main or therapeutic effect but still allows for the continuation of treatment (Wolf, 1989).

The aim of this chapter is to understand the safe administration of medicines.

LEARNING OUTCOMES

At the end of this chapter, the reader will be able to:

❑ Outline Nursing & Midwifery Council (NMC) guidance on administration of medicines.
❑ Outline causes of errors associated with the administration of medicines.

- Outline strategies to reduce the incidence of medication-related errors.
- Outline the essential principles of safe administration of medicines.
- Describe the administration of the correct medicine.
- Describe the administration of the correct dose.
- Describe the administration of the medicine at the right time/frequency.
- Describe the administration of medicines via the appropriate route.
- List circumstances where the prescription is correct, yet the route inappropriate for the patient.
- Discuss the evaluation of medicine effectiveness.
- Outline documentation issues associated with the administration of medicines.

NURSING & MIDWIFERY COUNCIL GUIDANCE ON ADMINISTRATION OF MEDICINES

In order to comply with the NMC (2008a) Code of Professional Conduct, nurses must ensure that their practice with regard to the administration of medicines is undertaken to reduce any associated risks to the patient and that the medicine is administered in a safe, systematic and efficient manner in line with local policies. Responsibilities also exist with regards to the procurement and storage of the medicine, as well as the ongoing assessment of its therapeutic effect.

Nurses do not only have to ensure that a medicine is administered as prescribed but also that the process is undertaken using their professional judgement. This is outlined in the NMC's statement below:

> *The administration of medicines is an important aspect of the professional practice of persons whose names are on the Council's register. It is not solely a mechanistic task to be performed in strict compliance with the written prescription of a medical practitioner. It requires thought and the exercise of professional judgement.*
>
> NMC (2008b)

The process of modernising the NHS has positively influenced new ways of working for registered nurses and has allowed for the development of advanced nurse practitioner roles with accompanying prescribing capabilities. Independent nurse prescribers are nurses or midwives who are trained to make a diagnosis and prescribe appropriate treatments that fall within their area of expertise and competence. They may also, in cases where a doctor has made an initial diagnosis, go on to prescribe or review and alter the medication prescribed, e.g. dosage, timing, frequency or route as part of the patients' clinical management plan (NMC, 2008b). This process places an even greater emphasis on professional accountability. Nurse prescribing is discussed in depth in Chapter 14.

CAUSES OF ERRORS ASSOCIATED WITH THE ADMINISTRATION OF MEDICINES

Errors can be defined as 'mistakes associated with medicines and intravenous infusions that are made during the prescription, transcription, dispensing and administration phases of medicine distribution' (Wolf, 1989).

It is thought that many incidents of medication error in the NHS often go undetected or unreported (DH, 2004); despite this the scale of the problem is large. In 2001, approximately 1200 people in England and Wales are thought to have died as a result of medication-related errors; this is an increase of 500% over the last decade (Scott, 2002). This increase may be related to the way in which medicine-related errors are now defined and subsequently reported. Between January 2005 and June 2006, NHS staff reported 59 802 medications safety incidents to the National Patient Safety Agency (NPSA); just over 80% of these errors occurred in acute, general or community hospital settings (NPSA, 2007a).

The vast majority of medicine administration errors are multifaceted and the result of system failures (Cohen & Shastay, 2008). However, much work has been undertaken to identify specific causes (O'Shea, 1999; DH, 2004; Preston, 2004). Some causes include:

- failure to identify the patient correctly;
- poor arithmetic skills and errors in dose calculation;
- illegible or inaccurate prescription;

- workload and workforce variation;
- poor clinical knowledge of medications;
- incorrect use of electronic devices;
- failure to work within organisational policy/procedure.

STRATEGIES TO REDUCE THE INCIDENCE OF MEDICATION-RELATED ERRORS

Most medication errors are preventable and to this effect various strategies have been devised to help reduce their incidence, including:

- the implementation of the clinical governance frameworks in all aspects of medicine administration, including increased reporting and learning (DH, 2000; NPSA, 2003);
- good practice frameworks, such as those presented by the NPSA;
- improving the skills and competence of all staff involved in the administration process through education and training.

Nurses must ensure that their practice is competent, informed, evidence based, risk assessed and performed in line with organisation procedure/policy. Nurses, as a central component of multidisciplinary care, also have a responsibility to ensure that other disciplines involved in the overall process of medicine administration are working with the same objective goals to achieve the best possible outcomes for the patient to provide a high standard of patient-focused care.

ESSENTIAL PRINCIPLES OF SAFE ADMINISTRATION OF MEDICATIONS

The effective and safe administration of medicines to patients requires a partnership between the various health professionals concerned, doctors, pharmacists and nurses (Dougherty & Lister, 2008). All members of this team should be working collaboratively to ensure that:

- medicines are stored appropriately prior to use (see Chapter 1);
- the right patient receives the correct medicine at the correct dose and formulation;

- the medicine is administered via the most appropriate route;
- the medicine is administered at the correct time, at the correct rate, for the correct duration of treatment.

PROCEDURE FOR PATIENT IDENTIFICATION

Reducing and, where possible, eliminating errors in the matching of patients with their care is central to improving patient safety in the NHS (NPSA, 2004). Over the 12-month period from February 2006 to January 2007, the NPSA received 24382 reports of patients being mismatched to their care (NPSA, 2007b). A prescription of a medicine is highly individualised, and the decision to prescribe the medicine for that particular patient will have been based on a holistic healthcare assessment, taking into account many factors, including past medical history, concurrent medication and allergy status. Taking these factors into account, the elements of risk posed to the patient should be minimal.

In order to maintain this low risk, the nurse must ensure that the patient is correctly identified prior to medicine administration. All hospital inpatients in acute settings must wear wristbands (also known as identity bands) with accurate details that correctly identify them and match them to their care (NPSA, 2005). Wristbands can be used in the medicine administration process to correctly identify a patient, by matching the prescription against the patient. This does not, however, exclude a nurse from using less formal verbal communication to compliment the identification process.

Since 2007, NHS organisations must only use patient wristbands that meet the NPSA's design requirements and only include the following patient identifiers:

- last name;
- first name;
- date of birth;
- NHS number (if the NHS number is not immediately available, a temporary number should be used until it is);
- first line of their address (only in Wales);

All patients must be given a wristband on their admission to a clinical area, and it must be worn at all times during the period of their inpatient stay. The NPSA also suggests that if a member of staff removes a wristband it is their responsibility to ensure that it is replaced. If this cannot be done immediately they must make alternative arrangements to allow for correct patient identification.

There may be circumstances where wearing an identification wristband may not be possible because of either a clinical condition or a treatment, for example in those who have severe burns, multiple invasive access points or certain dermatological conditions. In such circumstances, all healthcare professionals must use other means, such as verbal confirmation, of patient identification prior to undertaking any activity related to their care.

Some patients may refuse to wear a wrist band despite clear explanation of the risks of not doing so. Measures should be in place to formally assess and manage the risks associated with identifying these patients (NPSA, 2005). If these measures involve questioning patients about their name, address, date of birth, etc., nursing staff should be mindful that the process should maintain patient confidentiality.

NHS numbers versus local identifier numbers

Between June 2006 and the end of August 2008, the NPSA received over 1300 reports of incidents resulting from confusion and errors about patients' identifying numbers. Many of these involved duplication in local numbering systems, for example two patients having the same number or one patient having more than one number (NPSA, 2009). In order to minimise the risk associated with this practice, the NPSA issued the following statement:

By 18 September 2009, all NHS organisations in England and Wales that provide primary, secondary and all other types of care such as community pharmacy should take the following action:

- Use the NHS number as the national patient identifier or the NHS number as the national patient identifier in conjunction with a local hospital numbering system (where local hospital numbers are used they must be used alongside and not instead of the NHS number).

- Primary care organisations that have stopped issuing medical record cards should reinstate this practice and use it as a means of informing patients about their NHS numbers and encouraging them to use these where appropriate.

ADMINISTRATION OF THE CORRECT MEDICINE

Adverse events related to inappropriate medicine administration are made because:

- a prescription is written on the incorrect patient's chart/file;
- the prescription is ambiguous;
- the prescription is correct but the medicine is contraindicated by the patient's condition;
- the prescription is correct but the medicine is contraindicated by extraneous events or circumstances have changed, for example scheduled surgery/investigation;
- there is confusion with medicine nomenclature;
- there is a failure in checking the medicine correctly.

Even the most diligent nurse working within an organisation's medicine policy could potentially administer a medicine not intended for and possibly contraindicated if the prescription was written for the wrong patient. The only protective mechanism against this is the nurse's professional judgement, knowledge and good practice. This, in itself, may not prevent the error initially but can prevent it from translating into practice and causing harm to the patient. The following case demonstrates this:

Mr Bernard Jones has had a course of intravenous benzylpenicillin prescribed on a thrice daily basis, a prescription which was intended for Mrs Augustine Jones. The nurse prepares the medicine correctly and identifies Mr Jones against the prescription using his wristband. As she does so she confirms his date of birth and asks if he is allergic to anything, to which he responds 'Penicillin'.

Ambiguous prescriptions

Computerised prescription systems may have gone some way to reduce the risk of error associated with ambiguous scripts. These systems are, however, only available in some institutions. The

Royal Pharmaceutical Society of Great Britain (RPSGB) have stipulated the legal requirements that must be met when hand-writing a prescription and these are outlined in Box 6.1. However, these are often not followed universally by some medical staff; problems are predominantly related to illegible handwriting, which may be subject to misinterpretation by nursing staff. Jenkins *et al.* (1993) found that between 4 and 10% of inpatient prescriptions were illegible or ambiguous.

In all cases, it is the nurse's professional judgement that will prevent error. Knowledge of the indications for, the effects of and the pharmacokinetics of a particular agent, as well as the correct doses, will be required. Prescriptions should not be blindly followed, and any ambiguity should be questioned with the

---

Box 6.1 Guidelines for prescription writing

- Prescriptions should be written indelibly.
- Prescriptions should be dated, stating the full name and address of the patient.
- Prescriptions should be signed by the prescriber.
- The age and date of birth of the patient should preferably be stated.
- The unnecessary use of decimal points should be avoided.
- Quantities of 1 g or more should be written as 1 g, etc.
- Quantities less than 1 g should be written in milligrams (mg).
- Quantities less than 1 mg should be written in micrograms.
- If decimals are used, a zero should be written in front of the decimal point.
- Micrograms and nanograms should not be abbreviated.
- Dose and dose frequency should be stated; for 'as required' medicines a minimum dose interval should be specified.
- Drug names should not be abbreviated.
- Specific directions should be written in English, with the exception of some Latin abbreviation (as listed in the British National Formulary).

(BMA & RPSGB, 2009)

---

prescriber prior to administration. It is not acceptable to not administer a medicine just because the prescription is illegible or subject to misinterpretation; to do so, without making attempts to ascertain the correct prescription, would result in a failure in duty of care and be incongruent with the code of conduct (NMC 2008a).

Exclusion of contraindications

Nurses must employ their professional judgement in all cases of medicine administration, knowing the indications for, the pharmacokinetics of and the usual dosage of the medicine along with any side effects and contraindications (Trounce, 2000). Nurses should also be familiar with how pathophysiological processes can influence the actions or effects of a particular medicine.

Many nurses develop knowledge about medicine therapy and disease process through experience, particularly that of their specific speciality, but it would be impossible to possess knowledge of each specific medicine and its individual mode of action and potential side effects. Access to this information is available from specific medicine information guides, most notably the *British National Formulary* (BNF) [British Medical Association (BMA) & RPSGB, 2009]. If other medicine guides are used, the validity of these should be agreed with the pharmacy department. Collaborative working relationships with the pharmacist are also essential in providing nurses with the knowledge required to reduce the risk of adverse events.

All patients should be offered information and education about their therapy; discussing the medicines about to be administered can provide valuable information about side effects of, contraindications to and previous responses to therapy. Discussing therapy with the patient should be an integral component of informed consent and should be the standard practice in medicine administration.

Computerised systems/packages are available that contain an electronic patient prescription chart. In some circumstances, these can be linked to laboratory data such as blood results, etc. Whilst these systems do not prevent errors, particularly those associated with checking, they can be instrumental in minimising their occurrence, for example if an attempt is made to prescribe a medicine that is contraindicated by the patient's condition, pre-programmed warnings will ensue to prevent or give advice about that prescription.

Extraneous events and their influence on the medicine administration process can also expose the patient to risk. Patients' journeys through the healthcare system are often unpredictable, particularly in acute care. The following case demonstrates this:

> An insulin-dependent patient who is being starved pre-operatively for urgent surgery is prescribed 30 units of insulin on the morning of his operation (his usual morning dose). Administration of this amount of insulin in a starving patient may induce hypoglycaemia, particularly when metabolic processes are about to be altered.

Forward planning of a patient's medicine plan should be an essential component of care planning and a key component of multidisciplinary review. It is likely that some patients, particularly the elderly or those with complicated disease processes, are treated with a considerable number of medicines, therefore there may be some interaction or potentiation of the individual therapies. Nurses must have some awareness of these interactions. The nurse is assisted greatly in these circumstances by the pharmacist, with whom a good working relationship will enhance the safety of patient care (Trounce, 2000).

Problems with medicine nomenclature

European law requires the use of the recommended international non-proprietary name (rINN) for medicinal substances (BMA & RPSGB, 2009). In the UK, the British-approved name (BAN) has been used for some substances. Whilst there is some similarity between the two names, the previous BAN has been changed to correspond with the rINN. This is to avoid confusion and prevent error across the European states. An up-to-date list of these changes is available in the BNF (BMA & RPSGB, 2009).

Failure in medicine checking

For most medicine administrations, particularly those in hospitals, a single registered nurse is required to check the medicine. It is thought that single nurse administration will result in greater care being given, since the nurse is aware that he/she is solely responsible and accountable (Dougherty & Lister, 2008). What has not been debated in recent years is whether having two nurses in the roles of checker and giver promotes safer medicine administration, thus reducing the risk of administration errors (Preston, 2004). Research evidence does indicate that the incidence of errors in prescribing, preparing and administering injectable medicines is higher than for other forms of medicine (NPSA, 2007c). For this reason, wherever possible two NMC} registrants should check medication to be administered intravenously, one of whom should also be the registrant who then administers the intravenous medication (NMC, 2008b).

ADMINISTRATION OF THE CORRECT DOSE

Risks to patient safety regarding medicine dosage are usually related to:

- errors in calculating medicine dosage;
- confusion with dose measurements;
- ambiguous/incorrect prescriptions (see above).

Calculating medicine dosage

One of the components of medicines administration is calculating the correct dose of a medicine to administer. This process can range from a simple mathematical calculation to complex calculations involving conversions and formulae; it should be noted that there is no minimum maths qualification required by the NMC for nurses to enter training (Wilson, 2003).

Incorrect dose calculations are a major source of error in medicines administration (DH, 2004). Trim (2004) suggests that for over 10 years, studies have demonstrated nurses' lack of proficiency in drug-related calculations. Many reasons have been put forward for this, and numerical competency and many strategies have been explored to address the problem. Independent two-nurse checking is suggested as good practice by the NMC (2008b).

Scott (2002) argues that whatever the student nurses' level of mathematical competency at the start of training, they need to be progressively helped to work towards a level of numerical competency by regular structured revision. Additional testing of this competency under examination conditions before training is completed would ensure that a basic standard is reached for all practitioners. Banning (2006) argues that all nurses who prescribe or administer medicines should be assessed for mathematical competence. Many nurses use calculators to perform medicine calculations, but this should not act as a substitute for arithmetical knowledge and skill (NMC, 2008a,b). Preston (2004) questions whether nurses should be encouraged to predict a logical answer mentally before they proceed with their chosen method for calculating a medicine dosage.

To minimise the number of errors caused by miscalculating dose, volume or rate of administration, nurses must be familiar with and apply a number of mathematical formulae (Trim, 2004). Nurses should also be familiar with units of measurement and conversion formulae within these measurements. The International System of Units (SI) is the modern form of the metric system and is used universally in health care. Some useful SI units and conversion formulae are given in Box 6.2. Basic medicine calculations and formulae are illustrated in Appendix 6.1.

Box 6.2 SI unit conversions

Many calculations require different volumes or weights to be converted into the same unit or value. To convert larger units to smaller, the larger is multiplied:

- kilograms (kg) to grams (g) = kg × 1000;
- grams to milligrams (mg) = g × 1000;
- milligrams to micrograms (mcg) = mg × 1000;
- micrograms to nanograms (ng) = mcg × 1000;
- litres (L) to millilitres (ml) = L × 1000.

To convert smaller units to larger, the smaller is divided:

- grams to kilograms = g/1000;
- milligrams to grams = mg/1000;
- micrograms to milligrams = mcg/1000;
- nanograms to micrograms = ng/1000;
- millilitres to litres = ml/1000.

Confusion with dose measurements

Incorrect doses through errors in prescribing, for example 100 mg being written rather than 10 mg or micrograms being confused with milligrams, may easily lead to errors, as would ambiguity in the prescription, as outlined above. Again the nurse's professional judgement and clinical knowledge will be the overall factor in preventing errors of this nature.

Pharmacy advice or confirmation of the correct dosage using a resource such as the BNF (BMA & RPSGB, 2009) will help to avoid errors. Errors can also occur because of confusion between medicine doses, as some medicine can be formulated at different concentrations, for example the sedative propofol is available as a 1% or 2% formulation. Diligence in prescription checking and thorough knowledge of a medicine and its usual dose and regimens will prevent errors.

ADMINISTRATION OF THE CORRECT FORMULATION

Drugs are rarely administered solely as pure chemical substances but are almost always given in formulated preparations. These can vary from relatively simple solutions to complex drug delivery systems through the use of appropriate additives or excipients in the formulation to provide varied and specialised pharmaceutical functions (Aulton, 2001). Many formulations are designed to achieve a predictable therapeutic response and ensure that medicines or their active ingredient are delivered in the most effective way.

For example, this may be via the enteral route, i.e. a formulation that is designed to be absorbed via the gastrointestinal tract or via the parenteral route, in which medicines are administered intravenously. Different medicine formulations are listed in Appendix 6.2. Within each of these groups certain processes or ingredients are utilised to ensure that the pharmacokinetics are the most effective.

Some medicines are formulated in such a way that their pharmacokinetics differs even though the active ingredients are the same, for example medicines that are released at different rates into the gastrointestinal tract, such as modified-release preparations. To ensure safety in medicine administration, it is of paramount importance to ensure that the formulation administered is appropriate for the patient. Again it will be the nurse's knowledge and clinical judgement along with collaborative working relationships with the pharmacist that will assist in avoiding these errors.

Medicine formulations and enteral feeding tubes

Enteral feeding tubes provide a means of maintaining nutritional intake when oral intake is inadequate or when there is restricted access to the gastrointestinal tract. Although parenteral administration can be used and often guarantees 100% absorption, repeated subcutaneous, intravenous or intramuscular injections are associated with complications and are not suitable for long-term use. Consideration should be given to alternative routes of administration, e.g. transdermal, rectal or buccal.

However, the enteral feeding tube itself can also be used as a route of administration. The use of this route for medicine administration has increased significantly in primary and secondary care (White & Bradnam, 2008). It is important to ensure that when delivering medications via this route, the formulation is appropriate. It is not acceptable to assume that a medicine that can be given orally is appropriate for enteral tube administration.

ADMINISTRATION OF THE MEDICINE AT THE RIGHT TIME/FREQUENCY

To ensure the optimal therapeutic effects and benefits of a medication, it must be administered in a timely manner to coincide with the objectives outlined in the patient's clinical management/treatment plan. The manufacturer's recommendations about the medicine administration are important, for example some medicines need to be administered prior to or with food. To administer a medicine at the incorrect time may lead to adverse events such as multidosing and medicine toxicity.

There are many factors that influence a medicine being given at the right time. These can be related to:

- supply/availability;
- nursing time/workload constraints;
- correct regime prescription.

Medicine supply/availability

Nurses have a responsibility to ensure that their clinical area keeps adequate stocks of commonly used medicinal products. This can only be achieved through collaboration with the pharmacy department; regular stock level checks by the pharmacy department will ensure that levels do not fall and will allow for stock rotation such that short-dated products are used first and out-of-date products are removed from circulation.

Pharmacy staff, however, are frequently not aware of unplanned changes in medicine usage, and these changes must be noted by nursing staff and communicated to ensure that adequate supplies are maintained. The use of non-stock medicines must also be communicated. If a non-stock medicine is required, prompt and efficient ordering from the pharmacy department will avoid any unnecessary delay in administration. Emergency medicines, as appropriate, should always be kept as stock in clinical areas. These include medicines for the management of cardiac arrest and anaphylaxis, since any delay in administration could prove to be fatal.

The elimination half-life of a drug (the time taken to fall to half the original concentration) will determine the amount of time it takes a drug to reach its therapeutic level within the body and hence will determine the dosing interval or frequency of administration. The frequencies of drug administration are outlined in Appendix 6.3.

Nursing time/workload constraints

The average day in a clinical area is unpredictable, with workload and staffing being dynamic. These effects will influence the timing of medicine administration. Palese *et al.* (2009) suggest that many errors are caused by the interruptions to which the nurse is subjected during medicine rounds and suggests that one interruption occurs for every 3.2 medication administrations.

Hospital medicine rounds should be organised to avoid interruptions. This may include checking that all equipment that may be needed during the medicine round is on the trolley before commencing medicine administration, as are the most commonly used medicines. If at all possible one nurse should be responsible for medicine administration to a small group of patients. One nurse administering for 32 patients will still be finishing the medicine round when the next one is due to start. Medicine round times should also be organised to complement ward activity. For example, a number of medicines need to be taken before, with or after food, therefore coincidence with meal times may be beneficial.

Medicine administration by nurses in the community may not be subject to the same restraints, but likewise interruptions can and will occur. Appropriate workload planning can ensure that medicines are given at the correct time.

Self-medicating patients should also be educated to appreciate the importance of correct frequency and advised appropriately.

Correct prescription regime

Prescribers, particularly doctors, unfamiliar with the routine in a particular clinical area may need some assistance in planning drug regimes so that the dose frequency coincides with other care therapies/activities.

ADMINISTRATION OF MEDICINES VIA THE APPROPRIATE ROUTE

Medicines can be administered via a number of different routes, including:

- oral;
- enteral (via feeding tubes such as nasogastric and gastro/jejunostomy);
- topical (intranasal, eye drops, creams and ointments);
- transdermal;
- intradermal;
- subcutaneous;
- intramuscular;
- intravenous.

This list is not exhaustive; other routes of medicine administration may be used in specialist areas but are not covered in this text. These routes are discussed in Chapters 9, 10 and 12.

Ensuring that the patient receives a medicine via the right route is of paramount importance to maximise therapeutic effect and reduce the risk of adverse effect/reaction. Administration of an agent formulated for oral enteral use via the parenteral route can have catastrophic and possibly fatal outcomes for the patient. Incorrect intravenous administration of oral liquid medicines has resulted in three reported deaths between 2001 and 2004, and there have been reports of four incidents of harm or near misses between 1997 and 2004 (NPSA, 2007d).

Errors concerning administering a medicine via the incorrect route can occur because of:

- incorrect/ambiguous prescription (see above);
- lack of concentration during administration;
- confusion from multimedicine administrations, for example the critically ill patient receiving enteral and parenteral agents;
- similar equipment used for enteral and parenteral administrations.

As with all aspects of medicine administration, it is the knowledge and professional judgement of the nurse along with collaborative working relationships with pharmacists and prescribers that will prevent error.

Certain recommendations have been made to help minimise the errors regarding routes of administration (NPSA, 2007d).

CARE STRATEGIES TO MINIMISE INTERRUPTIONS TO THE MEDICINE ADMINISTRATION PROCESS

If a patient is receiving multiroute medicines, these should be delivered in 'route groups', for example prepare and administer the intravenous agents first, then wash hands and prepare and administer the oral medicines.

The NPSA recommends that only labelled oral/enteral syringes that cannot be connected to intravenous catheters or ports should be used to measure and administer oral liquid medicines (NPSA, 2007d) They also go on to recommend that any enteral feeding system should not contain ports that can be connected to intravenous syringes or that have end connectors that can be connected to intravenous or other parenteral lines.

Three-way taps and syringe tip adaptors should not be used in enteral feeding systems, as they allow connection design safeguards to be bypassed (NPSA, 2007d).

CIRCUMSTANCES WHERE THE PRESCRIPTION IS CORRECT, YET THE ROUTE INAPPROPRIATE FOR THE PATIENT

Just as nursing judgement is required when ascertaining if a medicine is appropriate for the patient, it is also required when establishing if the route of administration is the most appropriate. Sometimes this may seem obvious: a patient who is fasting pre surgery is prescribed their normal twice-daily oral furosemide on the morning of the operation. The nurse should question this and refer to the prescriber or the anaesthetic team. Is the medicine required? If so would it be more appropriate to administer it via the intravenous route?

More commonly, patients who are experiencing nausea and vomiting are prescribed oral medicines, where administration via this route will lead to ineffective drug delivery and in such instances parenteral administration would be more appropriate.

EVALUATION OF MEDICINE EFFECTIVENESS

Nurses are an integral, central component to multidisciplinary care, therefore they are best placed to evaluate the effectiveness of all aspects of care and treatment. This is particularly important with medicine therapy. Nurses also require, as a part of professional judgement, to be able to evaluate the effectiveness of a particular therapy in order to make balanced clinical decisions.

This evaluation explores not only the clinical effectiveness of a particular therapy in isolation but also how it affects that patient from a holistic perspective. For example, a patient who is commenced on a course of intravenous antibiotics for a post-operative wound infection may initially respond to therapy as indicated by improved wound healing, decrease in systemic temperature and a decrease in inflammatory markers. However, the patient's risk of subsequent infection is increased by intravenous access devices and phlebitis. Indications of this can be identified easily and quickly through holistic nursing assessment. Discussion of such findings at a multidisciplinary level will lead to enhanced care and improved patient outcomes.

Monitoring the effects of medicines is equally important in the community setting, as preventable medicine-related admissions to hospital are thought to be high and specifically related to certain medicine groups (Howard *et al.*, 2003).

Evaluating medicines effectiveness will include:

- comprehensive patient assessment, including measurement of vital signs;
- specific therapeutic drug monitoring, as indicated – whilst this is traditionally a doctor's domain, it will be incorporated in the assessment process;
- reporting adverse reactions via an organisation's clinical governance framework and possibly the yellow card framework as outlined in the BNF (BMA & RPSGB, 2009);
- patient education – patients should be advised about the intended effects of medicines as well as potential side effects and encouraged to monitor these and allowed to communicate their experiences of medicines.

DOCUMENTATION ISSUES ASSOCIATED WITH ADMINISTRATION OF MEDICINES

The underlying principle of documentation is to provide a record of patient care and treatment, and through this process improve communication as well as promote safety. Errors or omissions in nursing documentation in medicines administration could lead to potentially fatal errors.

All processes during medicine administration must be documented clearly as outlined by the NMC (NMC, 2007):

- This process must record discussions you have, the assessments you make, the treatment and medicines you give, and how effective these have been. If medications have been omitted the reasons for this and any subsequent actions taken should be recorded.
- You must ensure any entries you make in someone's paper records are clearly and legibly signed, dated and timed.
- You must ensure any entries you make in someone's electronic records are clearly attributable to yourself.

[Adapted from *The Code: Standards of Conduct, Performance and Ethics for Nurses and Midwives* (NMC, 2008a)]

CONCLUSION

This chapter has provided an overview to the principles of safe administration of medicines. NMC guidance has been discussed and causes of errors associated with the administration of medicines have been listed. Strategies to reduce the incidence of medication-related errors and the essential principles of safe administration of medicines have been outlined. The administration of the correct medicine at the correct dose, at the right time/frequency and via the appropriate route has been discussed. Circumstances where the prescription is correct, yet the route inappropriate for the patient, have been listed. The evaluation of medicine effectiveness and documentation issues associated with administration of medicines have been outlined.

APPENDIX 6.1 BASIC DRUG CALCULATIONS AND FORMULAE

To calculate infusion rates for larger volumes of fluid via gravity administration sets

To administer fluid volumes over a specified time a gravitational flow administration set may be used, which requires the infusion rate to be administered as 'drops per minute'. To calculate this, the number of drops per millilitre for the specific set must be ascertained – this is usually identified on the packaging. Generally, crystalloid administration sets operate at 20 drops per millilitre (d/ml) and blood (large-bore) sets operate at 15 d/ml.

To calculate the infusion rate in drops per minute the following formula is applied:

volume required/duration (h) × set value (d/ml)/min (60)

Illustration

Patient A is prescribed 1000 ml of Hartmann's solution to be administered over 6 h using an administration set with a value of 20 d/ml:

$$1000/6 \times 20/60 = 55 \, \text{d/min}$$

To calculate larger-volume infusion rates when administered via an electronic volumetric pump, the rate will be set in millilitres per hour

To calculate ml to be delivered/infusion time, the following formula is applied.

Illustration

Dextrose saline 500 ml is to be administered over 3 h:

$$500/3 = 166 \text{ ml per hour}$$

To calculate a required drug volume from stock strength

This is a common calculation as many prescribed doses are smaller than the available preparation. In some drugs, the stock concentration may depend on the volume of diluent. This is often the case in reconstituting antibiotics. The following formula is applied:

amount required/stock strength × stock volume

or more simply

what you want/what you have got × volume

Illustration

Cefuroxime 300 mg (which is available as a 750 mg vial) is required from a reconstituted vial of 300 mg in 10 ml:

$$300/750 \times 10 = 4 \text{ ml}$$

Unless contraindicated, it may be useful to reconstitute the drug in a volume of fluid that makes it easier to calculate a mentally logical answer. For example, by diluting the cefuroxime above in 10 ml the nurse is aware that half the volume will contain 375 mg of the drugs, thus a mental logical calculation identifies that just under half the volume is required.

Calculating weight-related doses

Occasionally, and particularly in paediatrics, drugs are prescribed based on the patient's body weight. The prescription may be expressed as a volume (millilitres per kilogram, ml/kg), or weight (milligrams per kilogram, mg/kg). The following formula is applied:

$$\text{prescribed volume} \times \text{body weight}$$

or

$$\text{prescribed dose} \times \text{body weight}$$

Illustrations
A patient with sepsis is prescribed 3 mg/kg of gentamycin intravenously. The patient's weight is 75 kg:

$$3 \times 75 = 225 \text{ mg}$$

A child weighing 4.5 kg is being fluid resuscitated in the emergency department. Local policy for this is 20 ml/kg:

$$20 \times 4.5 = 90 \text{ ml}$$

Calculating drug concentrations (mg/ml) where the drug is expressed as a percentage

Some drugs are presented in a percentage concentration (for example, lidocaine, calcium chloride and dextrose in solution).

The expression refers to grams per 100 ml, so a 1% solution would be 1 g per 100 ml and a 50% solution would be 50 g per 100 ml. The volume always remains constant.

Illustration:
How many mg/ml are there in 2% lignocaine?
2% = 2 g in 100 ml, which is the equivalent of 2000 mg in 100 ml (calculated using SI conversion formulae):

$$2000 \text{ mg}/100 \text{ ml} = 20 \text{ mg/ml}$$

Once a mg/ml concentration has been calculated, further formulae such as dose or stock strength × volume may be necessary to calculate the volume required.

Concentrations from weight-to-volume ratios

Some drugs are expressed as a weight-to-volume ratio (such as adrenaline and noradrenaline). These could be expressed as 1:1000 or 1:10000.

The expression is similar to a percentage except that the weight remains constant (1 g) and the volume differs. The volume is in millilitres, therefore:

- adrenaline 1:10000 = 1 g in 10000 ml;
- noradrenaline 1:1000 = 1 g in 1000 ml.

Illustration

How many milligrams are there in 1 ml of adrenaline 1:10000?

$$1:10\,000 = 1\,g\ in\ 10\,000\ ml$$

which is the equivalent of 1000 mg in 10000 ml (calculated using SI conversion formulae):

$$1000/10\,000 = 0.1\,mg/ml$$

(which can be converted into micrograms per millilitre using SI conversion formulae).

Once a mg/ml concentration has been calculated, further formulae such as dose or stock strength × volume may be necessary to calculate the volume required.

[Adapted from Higgins D. (2005) Drug calculations. *Nursing Times* **101**(46): 24–25; with permission.]

APPENDIX 6.2 DRUG FORMULATIONS

The absorption patterns of drugs will vary considerably between one another as well as between each potential route of administration. Dosage forms are designed to present the drug in a suitable form for maximal absorption and delivery to its target site, depending on the selected route of administration.

Enteral formulations

Tablets

These are the most convenient and acceptable forms of oral medication (Hopkins, 1999). Tablets consist of the active ingredient with a filler starch, a substance that will disintegrate in the gastro-intestinal tract along with binding and lubricating agents. These additional agents are known as excipients (Galbraith *et al.*, 1999).

If any of the above agents taste unpleasant, a sugar or film coating may be used to improve patient compliance.

Enteric-coated formulations

Some tablets have a coating that will allow passage of the drug unchanged into the small intestine, as the active ingredient or any of the excipients may be irritant to the gastric mucosa. These tablets should not be split, crushed or chewed. Capsules can also be formulated with the same properties, and these are termed gastro-resistant.

Capsules

The active ingredient is contained within a gelatine case. In the case of powders, particularly antibiotics, a hard case is used, but soft-shelled capsules can be used for agents suspended in oil. Capsules should be swallowed whole, and no attempt should be made to open or split the capsule (Hopkins, 1999).

Modified-release formulations

Some enteral tablets and capsules, particularly those that have short half-lives, are formulated to release the active ingredient over a prolonged period of time. The chemical processes that control the rate of release differ, often from company to company. Modified-release drugs should be swallowed whole, and no attempt should be made to open or alter the formulation prior to administration.

Liquid formulations

These are used in all aspects of health care but are particularly useful in paediatrics, to make the drug more palatable and tolerable. They are also of great use in patients where gastrointestinal access is obtained via a feeding tube. If a drug is insufficiently soluble in water, alcoholic solutions can be used – these are termed elixirs.

Sublingual formulations

Drugs can be absorbed through the mucosa of the mouth, which avoids the mixing (and potential altering) of a drug with food, fluid and gastric juices. Drugs administered by this route can also be absorbed into the bloodstream without first passing through the liver (by-passing the hepatic first-pass effect). These drugs should not be swallowed but rather retained in the sublingual or buccal pouch. Specific patient education will be required to max-imise therapeutic effect.

Rectal formulations

Administering a drug in a rectal formulation may have signifi-cant benefits, most notably good and often slow absorption and the avoidance of the hepatic first-pass effect. Suppositories contain the active ingredient in a base that melts in response to an increase in temperature. Enemas tend to be fluid based and are formulated either to distend the bowel or to soften faeces. Local anti-inflammatory drugs can also have direct effect. Pessaries are formulated in a similar fashion but are intended for vaginal use.

Parenteral formulations

Inhaled formulations

These formulations use the surface area of the lung for absorption and are often delivered as aerosols, which can provide a rapid response to therapy. In some therapies, such as bronchodilatory drugs, the delivery of the active ingredient to target cells can reduce dose requirements and minimise systemic effects (Hopkins, 1999). Patient education and the possible use of drug delivery aids such as volumatic spacers are of paramount impor-tance in maximising therapeutic effect.

Injectable drugs

Some drugs are formulated as a solution or suspension for inject-able use via the intradermal, subcutaneous, intramuscular or intravenous route. These formulations are produced as sterile solutions and can be given, if licensed, via other routes, for example actrapid insulin, normally given subcutaneously, can also be given intravenously in some acute situations. Nurses administering the medicine must ensure that the injectable drug is licensed for the particular route that is to be used. Injectable drugs can be water based or lipid based; some may require aseptic reconstitution with a diluent prior to administration to facilitate delivery. Injectable drugs are supplied as single-dose ampoules although multi-dose vials, with the addition of preservatives, are also available.

Topical preparations

These drugs are formulated for local or protective action and must not be ingested. Drug presentation may be an oil- or water-based cream/liniment. Trans-dermal patches, which contain a reservoir of a drug that can be released at a controlled rate, are becoming more popular in primary and secondary care.

APPENDIX 6.3 DRUG FREQUENCIES

Whilst abbreviations in drug prescribing are best avoided, it is recognised that some Latin abbreviations are used when prescribing. These abbreviations and their meanings are outlined below.

Abbreviation	Latin	Translation
o.d.	Omni die	Once per day
b.d.	Bis die	Twice per day
t.d.s.	Ter die sumendus	Three times daily
q.d.s.	Quarter die sumendus	Four times daily
a.c.	Ante cibum	Before food
o.m.	Omi mane	Every morning
o.n.	Omi nocte	Every night
p.c.	Post cibum	After food
p.r.n.	Pro re nata	As required
q.q.h.	Quarta quaque hora	Every 4 h
Stat		Immediately

Each prescription should be written with a time for administration.
Adapted from BMA & RPSGB (2009).

REFERENCES

Aulton M (2001) *Pharmaceutics: The Science of Dosage Form Design*, 2nd edn. Blackwell Publishing, Oxford.

Banning M (2006) Medication errors: professional issues and concerns. *Nurs Older People* **18**(3): 27–32.

British Medical Association & Royal Pharmaceutical Society of Great Britain (BMA & RPSGB) (2009) *British National Formulary*. BMJ Publishing Group Ltd, London, and RPS Publishing, London.

Cohen H, Shastay AD (2008) Getting to the root of medication errors. *Nursing* **38**(12): 39–47.

Department of Health (DH) (2000) *An Organisation with a Memory*. The Stationary Office, London.

Department of Health (DH) (2004) *Building a Safer NHS for Patients: Improving Medication Safety*. Crown Copyright, London. Available at www.doh.gov.uk/buildsafenhs/medicationsafety [accessed in June 2009].

Dougherty L, Lister S (2008) *The Royal Marsden Hospital Manual of Clinical Nursing Procedures*, 7th edn. Wiley-Blackwell, Oxford.

Galbraith A, Bullock S, Mainias E, Hunt B, Richards A (1999) *Fundamentals of Pharmacology: a Text for Nurses and Health Professionals*. Pearson Prentice-Hall, Harlow.

Hopkins SJ (1999) *Drugs and Pharmacology for Nurses*, 13th edn. Churchill Livingstone, London.

Howard RL, Avery AJ, Howard PD, Partridge M (2003) Investigation into the reasons for preventable drug related admissions to a medical admissions unit: observational study. *Qual Safe Health Care* **12**: 280–285.

Jenkins D, Cairns C, Barber N (1993) The quality of written inpatient prescriptions. *Int J Pharm Pract* **2**(3): 176–179.

National Patient Safety Agency (NPSA) (2003) *Seven Steps to Patient Safety for Primary Care*. NPSA, London.

National Patient Safety Agency (NPSA) (2004) *Right Patient – Right Care*. NPSA, London.

National Patient Safety Agency (NPSA) (2005) *Safer Practice Notice 11: Wristbands for Hospital Inpatients Improves Safety*. NPSA, London.

National Patient Safety Agency (NPSA) (2007a) *Safety in Doses, Improving Medication Safety Within the NHS*. NPSA, London.

National Patient Safety Agency (NPSA) (2007b) *Standardising Wristbands Improves Patient Safety*. NPSA, London.

National Patient Safety Agency (NPSA) (2007c) *Patient Safety Alert 20: Promoting Safer Use of Injectable Medicines*. NPSA, London.

National Patient Safety Agency (NPSA) (2007d) *Patient Safety Alert 19: Promoting Safer Measurement and Administration of Liquid Medicines via Oral and Other Enteral Routes*. NPSA, London.

National Patient Safety Agency (NPSA) (2009) *Risk to Patient Safety of Not Using the NHS Number as the National Identifier for all Patients*. NPSA, London.

Nursing & Midwifery Council (NMC) (2007) *Record Keeping Advice Sheet*. Available at www.nmc-uk.org/aDisplayDocument.aspx?documentID=4008 [accessed in June 2009].

Nursing & Midwifery Council (NMC) (2008a) *The Code: Standards of Conduct, Performance and Ethics for Nurses and Midwives*. NMC, London.

Nursing & Midwifery Council (NMC) (2008b) *Standards for Medicines Management*. NMC, London.

O'Shea E (1999) Factors contributing to medication errors: a literature review. *J Clin Nurs* **8**: 496–504.

Palese A, Sartor A, Costaperaria G, Bresadola V (2009) Interruptions during nurses' drug rounds in surgical wards: observational study. *J Nurs Manage* **2**: 185–192.

Preston RM (2004) Drug errors and patient safety: the need for a change in practice. *Br J Nurs* **13**: 72–78.

Scott H (2002) Increasing number of patients are being given wrong drugs. *Br J Nurs* **11**(1): 4.

Trim J (2004) Clinical skills: a practical guide to working out drug calculations. *Br J Nurs* **13**(10): 602–606.

Trounce J (2000) *Clinical Pharmacology for Nurses*. Churchill Livingstone, London.

White R, Bradnam V (2008) *Handbook of Drug Administration via Enteral Feeding Tubes*. PhP Pharmaceutical Press, London.

Wilson A (2003) Nurses maths: researching a practical approach. *Nurs Stand* **17**(47): 33–36.

Wolf ZR (1989) Medication errors and nursing responsibility. *Holist Nurs Pract* **4**(1): 8–17.

Wright K (2009) Supporting the development of calculating skills in nurses. *Br J Nurs* **7**: 399–402.

7 | Medication Errors

Ruth Endacott

INTRODUCTION

According to the National Patient Safety Agency [National Patient Safety Agency (NPSA), 2003], 'Every day more than a million people are treated safely and successfully in the NHS; this treatment often includes the use of medicines.' However, advances in the development and regulation of medicines also mean that a single drug may be available in a number of different forms, with variable actions (for example, long or short acting) and a number of different trade names. Patients are also increasingly likely to be taking medication for more than one chronic condition, and these medications may be prescribed, dispensed and administered by a number of different health professionals. These complexities increase the potential for medication error.

The term medication error has been defined by the NPSA as follows:

> A medication error *is any preventable event that may cause or lead to inappropriate medication use or patient harm while the medication is in the control of health professional, patient or consumer.*
>
> [Department of Health (DH), 2004]

Medication errors may occur at any stage of the medication process and hence involve prescribing and ordering; dispensing and distribution; preparation and administration; labelling, packaging and drug nomenclature; communications and education; or use and monitoring of treatment. Most medication errors do not result in harm to the patient. However, the use of any medicine carries an inherent risk and the majority of medicines have the potential to cause harm if used inappropriately or incorrectly.

Medication errors can result in hospital admission or readmission; Witherington and colleagues (2008) reviewed the records of

108 patients aged over 75 who were readmitted as an emergency within 28 days of discharge from hospital. They found that 38% (41) of readmissions were related to medications and over 60% (25) of medication-related readmissions were preventable.

LEARNING OUTCOMES
At the end of the chapter, the reader will be able to:

❏ Discuss the most common types of medication error.
❏ Discuss factors increasing the risk of medication error.
❏ Outline strategies to reduce medication errors.

COMMON TYPES OF MEDICATION ERROR
Medication incidents tend to be classified according to the actual or potential harm that results (see Figure 7.1). The type of incident indicates the actions to be taken.

In addition to the classification in Figure 7.1, medication incidents can be the result of action omitted or action taken – errors of omission or errors of commission.

Errors of omission
There are three common types of omission error:

* omitting adverse drug reactions when taking or recording the patient's history;

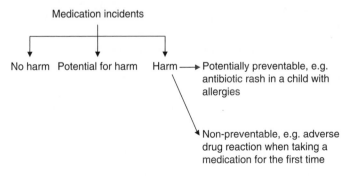

Fig 7.1 Types of medication incident. Reproduced under the terms of the click-use licence

- omitting drug allergies when taking or recording the patient's history;
- omitting to administer medications.

Failing to record adverse drug reactions or drug allergies are identified as common errors in patient documentation (Medical Protection Society, 2008), but medication administration also involves monitoring the patient to determine whether or not the medication is working and to detect any unexpected response. In many healthcare settings, prescribing, administering and monitoring the effects of medication will be undertaken by different health professionals, emphasising the need for clear verbal and written communication.

Failure to administer prescribed medications (medication omissions) has been identified in a number of studies. A study undertaken in medical and surgical wards across four NHS Trusts in England identified that nearly 80% of patients (129/162) missed at least one dose of a medication, with a significant relationship between length of stay and the likelihood of missing medications (Warne *et al.*, in press). Other studies report that medication errors are more likely in the first 48 h after admission (Ho *et al.*, 1997; NPSA, 2007) or the first 48 h after a drug is prescribed (Ho *et al.*, 1997).

Errors of commission

The four main errors of commission in medication management occur during:

- *medication prescribing*: this has been found across the range of care settings, including general practice (Rubin *et al.*, 2003), hospital inpatients (Dean *et al.*, 2002) and intensive care units (ICUs) (Ridley *et al.*, 2004);
- *medication labelling*: for example of infusion syringes for intravenous use (Wheeler *et al.*, 2008);
- *transfer of prescriptions to a new medication record*: in one study, 26% of all prescriptions on ICU transfer reports contained errors (Perren *et al.*, 2008);
- *drug calculations*: these have been identified as a key factor in neonatal and paediatric medication errors (NPSA, 2009).

FACTORS INCREASING THE RISK OF MEDICATION ERROR

Organisational factors

The 'Swiss cheese model' (Reason, 1997) of system failure can help us understand how medication errors can occur. Each slice of cheese represents a safeguard against error; whilst each 'slice', or safeguard, should be intact, in reality the slices are full of holes. As the number of safeguards increases, it becomes less likely that the 'holes' in the system will align sufficiently to allow an error to occur. Figure 7.2 identifies some of the layers of defence against medication error.

There are two reasons for holes opening up in the layers of defence: active failures and latent conditions (Reason, 1990). Active failures result from unsafe practices of the people working with a system, for example the doctor failing to check for drug

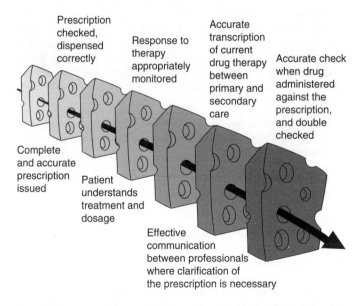

Fig 7.2 Swiss cheese model of error prevention: some layers of defence against medication error (DH, 2004; with permission)

allergies or the pharmacist failing to identify an incorrect dose on a prescription. Latent conditions are the aspects of the systems, such as the resources available and medication policies, which, either alone or in combination with an active failure, can result in error. Examples of latent conditions include:

- the lack of a computerised prescribing system with in-built systems to highlight an erroneous prescription;
- the absence of an effective communication system between primary and secondary care;
- the absence of system checks to ensure that drugs with similar names or packaging are not wrongly administered.

In a further development of his work, Reason (2004) suggests that early identification of potential for error can be assisted using the 'three buckets' model. The three buckets contain factors relating to: (1) the individual undertaking the task (lack of knowledge, fatigue, inexperience and feeling under the weather), (2) the context in which the task is completed (distractions, interruptions and lack of time) and (3) the task itself (lack of cueing from preceding steps). These factors can be applied to any aspect of the medication management process from prescribing through to administration and monitoring for the therapeutic and non-therapeutic effects of the medication. Consider the following scenario:

It is 14:00 h in a busy medical ward; there are a number of patients waiting to be discharged and two patients in the Emergency Department waiting for a bed. The medications due at 14:00 h have not yet been administered. The nurse in charge asks the newly qualified registered nurse, who has just come back from a week's leave and just commenced the shift, to 'do the drug round'.

Applying Reason's model of error potential to this scenario, the 'buckets' would appear to be fairly full: the nurse is inexperienced, does not know the patients and is already under pressure as the drugs are late and the ward is busy. Similar scenarios could be written to depict the busy context in which medications are sometimes prescribed. In these situations, Reason's model can provide a useful audit of error potential to identify factors that could be addressed to improve the safety of medication administration.

Type of medication

Review of medication errors highlights a particular problem with the preparation and administration of intravenous medications (Cousins *et al.*, 2005; NPSA, 2007).

Children and neonates are also at particular risk of medication error (NPSA, 2007, 2009). The most common errors in these age groups are administration of the wrong dose or strength of a medication as a result of inaccurate drug calculation (NPSA, 2009). There are a number of factors that increase the complexity of drug calculations with children and neonates (NPSA, 2009):

- Calculations are usually based on the age and weight of the child.
- Outside of paediatric hospitals, medication doses may require administration of part of a tablet or ampoule intended for adult use.
- Liquid preparations, commonly used for younger children, are often available in more than one strength.
- Medications sometimes require the conversion of doses from milligrams to micrograms – one of the most common paediatric medication errors is ten-fold dosing errors.

STRATEGIES TO REDUCE MEDICATION ERRORS

The approaches taken by Reason (1997, 2004) to understand how errors arise (for example, the Swiss cheese and three buckets models) emphasise the need to review systems in order to limit the occurrence of errors and minimise their impact. As a result, much of the effort in health services is directed at understanding the conditions under which medications are prescribed, dispensed and administered and how to adapt those conditions to reduce errors.

In the UK, the Chief Medical Officer's report to Ministers in 2000, *An Organisation with a Memory* (DH, 2000), proposed a strategy for improving care by reporting and learning from adverse events. The report specifically focused on the need to move from 'passive learning', where lessons to be learnt are identified but not carried through to practice, to 'active learning', where lessons learnt are subsequently embedded in the culture of the healthcare setting. Strategies to reduce errors in the prescribing, dispensing and administration of medications are specifically addressed in an implementation report: *Building a safer NHS: improving medication safety* (DH, 2004). Table 7.1 identifies some of the key risks of medication error and measures to reduce risk.

Medication incidents where there is potential for harm but no harm has actually occurred are classified as a 'near miss' or 'close call'. A quality improvement initiative in the USA changed terminology from 'close call' to 'good catch' and found an increase in reporting of these types of errors (Mick *et al.*, 2007),

Table 7.1 Factors increasing risk of error and strategies to improve medication safety when prescribing and administering medications

Risk of error	Strategies to reduce risk
Inadequate knowledge of the patient and their clinical condition	Regular review of long-term repeat prescribing
Poor history taking	Implementation of electronic prescribing
Inadequate knowledge of the medication	Implementation of electronic care records
Calculation errors	Clear treatment plans, developed and reviewed in consultation with all professionals involved in the patient's care
Illegible handwriting	
Drug name confusion	
Failure to clarify an ambiguous or badly written prescription	Double checking of all complex medication calculations
	Clear drug administration procedures, relevant to the setting in which medicines are administered
	Appropriate training for all staff involved in medication administration
	Checking with patients when medicines are prescribed, dispensed and administered
	Providing patients with the opportunity to ask questions about their medicines
	Safeguards built into electronic systems to prevent 'juxtaposition' errors

Adapted from DH (2004).

emphasising the benefits of shifting from a 'name, blame and shame' approach.

Following extensive review of medication errors, the NPSA (2007) proposed seven key steps to improve medication safety:

- Increase reporting and learning from medication incidents.
- Implement NPSA safer medication practice recommendations.
- Improve staff skills and competences.
- Minimise dosing errors.
- Ensure medicines are not omitted.
- Ensure the correct medicines are given to the correct patients.
- Document patients' medicine allergy status.

Electronic prescribing

One strategy to minimise medication errors is the use of electronic systems for prescribing, dispensing and administering medications. These systems are discussed more fully in Chapter 5. Electronic systems can reduce errors, although the evidence demonstrates variable success – one drawback is the reduced opportunities for face-to-face discussion about patient medication between nurses, doctors, pharmacist and the patient (Barber *et al.*, 2007).

CONCLUSION

Medication errors happen as a result of a number of complex and often inter-related factors. A number of strategies have been developed to improve recognition of situations in which medication error is more likely and to prevent errors occurring. It is important to identify which of these factors and strategies are present in your own practice setting.

REFERENCES

Barber N, Cornford T, Klecun E (2007) Qualitative evaluation of an electronic prescribing and administration system. *Qual Saf Health Care* **16**: 271–278.

Cousins DH, Sabatier B, Begue D, *et al.* (2005) Medication errors in intravenous drug preparation and administration: a multicentre audit in the UK, Germany and France. *Qual Saf Health Care* **14**: 190–195.

Dean B, Schachter M, Vincent C, Barber N (2002) Prescribing errors in hospital inpatients: their incidence and clinical significance. *Qual Saf Health Care* **11**: 340–344.

Department of Health (DH) (2000) *An Organisation with a Memory: Report of an Expert Group on Learning from Adverse Events in the NHS Chaired by the Chief Medical Officer*. The Stationery Office, London.

Department of Health (2004) *Building a Safer NHS for Patients: Improving Medication Safety*. The Stationery Office, London.

Ho CYW, Dean BS, Barber ND (1997) When do medication administration errors happen to hospital inpatients? *Int J Pharm Pract* **5**: 91–96.

Medical Protection Society (2008) *MPS Guide to Good Records*. Medical Protection Society, London.

Mick JM, Wood GL, Massey RL (2007) The good catch program: increasing potential error reporting. *J Nurs Adm* **37**(11): 499–503.

National Patient Safety Agency (NPSA) (2003) *Seven Steps to Patient Safety. A Guide for NHS Staff*. NPSA, London.

National Patient Safety Agency (NPSA) (2007) *The Fourth Report from Patient Safety Observatory. Safety in Doses: Medication Incidents in the NHS*. NPSA, London.

National Patient Safety Agency (NPSA) (2009) *Review of Patient Safety for Children and Young People*. NPSA, London.

Perren A, Conte P, de Bitonti N, Limono C, Merlani P (2008) From the ICU to the ward: cross-checking of the physician's transfer report by intensive care nurses. *Intens Care Med* **34**: 2054–2061.

Reason J (1990) *Human Error*. Cambridge University Press, Cambridge.

Reason J (1997) *Managing the Risks of Organisational Accidents*. Ashgate, Aldershot.

Reason J (2004) Beyond the organisational accident: the need for 'error wisdom' on the frontline. *Qual Saf Health Care* **13**(Suppl II): ii28–ii33.

Ridley SA, Booth SA, Thompson CM (2004) Prescription errors in UK critical care units. *Anaesthesia* **59**: 1193–2000.

Rubin G, George A, Chinn DJ, Richardson C (2003) Errors in general practice: development of an error classification and pilot study of a method for detecting errors. *Qual Saf Health Care* **12**: 443–447.

Warne S, Endacott R, Chamberlain W, *et al.* (in press) Non-therapeutic omission of medications in acutely ill patients. *Nurs Crit Care* (accepted for publication July 2009).

Wheeler DW, Degnan BA, Schmi JS, Burnstein RM, Menon DK, Gupta AK (2008) Variability in the concentrations of intravenous drug infusions prepared in a critical care unit. *Intens Care Med* **34**: 1441–1447.

Witherington EMA, Pirzada OM, Avery AJ (2008) Communication gaps and readmissions to hospital for patients aged 75 years and older: observational study. *Qual Saf Health Care* **17**(1): 71–75.

Basic Pharmacology of Common Medications

8

Gareth Walters

INTRODUCTION

Pharmacology explains how drugs interact with the systems of the human body (Neal, 2005). The purpose of this chapter is to provide an introduction to the basic pharmacology of some of the medications currently used in the healthcare setting. If required, a more detailed account can be found elsewhere, e.g. *British National Formulary* (BNF).

The aim of this chapter is to understand the basic pharmacology of common medications.

LEARNING OUTCOMES

At the end of this chapter, the reader will be able to:

❏ Discuss medications commonly used in cardiovascular disease.
❏ Outline medications acting on the kidneys.
❏ Discuss medications commonly used to treat infections.
❏ Discuss medications commonly used to treat pain and inflammation.

MEDICATIONS COMMONLY USED IN CARDIOVASCULAR DISEASE

Drugs acting on the cardiovascular system can be categorised into:

- drugs used for hypertension;
- drugs used for cardiac arrhythmias;
- drugs that treat heart failure;
- drugs used for ischaemic heart disease.

Drugs used for *hypertension* lower the systemic blood pressure in a number of ways. Blood pressure is product of cardiac output (CO) and total peripheral vascular resistance (TPR):

$$blood\ pressure = CO \times TPR$$

Drugs that lower CO by having a negatively inotropic effect on the heart (reduce the forcefulness of the heart muscle contraction) or reduce peripheral vascular resistance (by increasing the diameter of blood vessels) will reduce the systemic blood pressure. Additionally, drugs that act on the central nervous system (CNS) to reduce neural drive to the heart and arterial tree, and drugs that reduce the total circulating blood volume (by excreting water and/or sodium) can have the same effect.

Cardiac arrhythmias are variations in the heartbeat from the normal 'sinus rhythm' of the heart. The heartbeat starts when electrical impulses generated in the sinus node of the right atrium of the heart (see Figure 8.1) spread sequentially through the heart muscle via the atrioventricular (AV) node to the ventricle, in order that the ventricular muscle can contract to produce a single normal heart beat. 'Sinus rhythm' describes the repetitive heartbeat that is produced from the sinus node. It is regular, at a rate between 60 and 100 beats per minute.

Cardiac arrhythmias can originate in any part of the heart's electrical conducting system. They are usually due to over-excitability of the heart and are often fast (tachycardias: >100 beats per minute) but can also be slow (bradycardias: <60 beats per minute). Disorders that cause over-excitability are ischaemic heart disease (for example immediately post-myocardial infarction), drugs (such as caffeine and salbutamol) and electrolyte abnormality (such as hyperkalaemia).

Drugs used to treat arrhythmias act on the parts of the conducting system that are responsible for generation of the arrhythmia, usually to block or delay conduction. However, disease in the electrical conduction system (from ischaemic heart disease or cardiomyopathy) sometimes causes delay in conduction to produce bradycardic arrhythmias (heart block), and drugs here are used to increase electrical conduction.

In a normally functioning heart the CO, i.e. the amount of blood passing through the left ventricle into the systemic circulation each minute in litres per minute, is the product of the stroke volume (SV, the amount of blood ejected by the ventricle in each contraction, usually 80 ml) and the heart rate (beats/min):

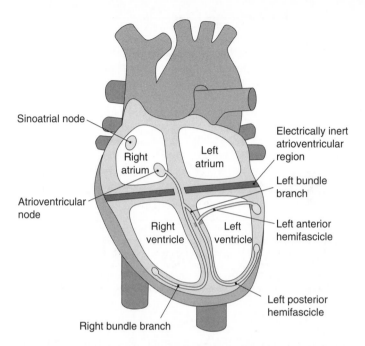

Fig 8.1 Conduction system of the heart. The diagram shows the spread of electrical conduction through the heart from the sinoatrial (SA) node via the atrioventricular (AV) node to the ventricles. Arrhythmias arising above the ventricle are called 'supraventricular'. Reproduced from Morris F, *et al. ABC of Clinical Electrocardiography*, 2nd edn, copyright 2008 with permission of Blackwell Publishing Ltd

$$CO\,(l/min) = SV\,(ml) \times heart\,rate\,(beats/min)$$

The SV in turn is proportional to the preload (the amount of blood entering the right side of the heart from the systemic circulation, also in litres per minute). For example, if the circulating volume is low, due to dehydration the preload will be low. It then follows from this rule that the SV will also be low. Thus, if the heartrate is constant, the CO will also be low (equal to the SV).

Starling's law suggests that preload and CO are directly proportional, up to an optimal preload value, and then as preload

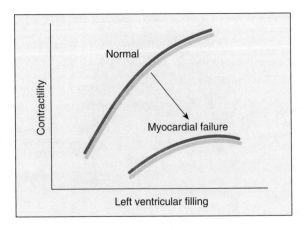

Fig 8.2 Starling's law. Preload and cardiac output are directly proportional up to an optimal preload, and then cardiac output starts to plateau before falling later on. In heart failure the myocardial contractility (strength of contraction) is much less for a given filling pressure. Reproduced from Gray H, Dawkins K, Morgan J, Simpson I, *Cardiology Lecture Notes*, 5th edn, copyright 2008, with permission of Blackwell Publishing Ltd

continues to increase (in states of fluid overload) the CO begins to fall (see Figure 8.2). In *heart failure* (which is defined as poor CO due to heart disease), fluid overload is common and preload is very high. This is what limits the CO. Drugs in heart failure reduce the preload by dilating blood vessels around the heart and also by reducing the circulating volume by diuresis.

Additionally in heart failure, the contractility of the heart (particularly of the left ventricle) is impaired by disease of the ventricular muscle (myocardium). This can be due to a variety of reasons, commonly ischaemic heart disease, heart valve disease or arrhythmia. This means that the SV (and thus CO) is reduced because the myocardium does not generate enough force to expel large volumes of blood. High preload and poor contractility cause fluid overload, particularly in the legs and on the lungs (pulmonary oedema). Drugs in heart failure can increase the contractility of the myocardium (positive inotropism) and reduce peripheral resistance to enhance the CO.

The term *ischaemic heart disease* describes the disorder caused by narrowing of the coronary arteries (coronary atherosclerosis). Ageing, smoking, hypertension and raised plasma cholesterol levels are all risk factors for damage to the lining of the artery wall (endothelium). This prompts the formation of cholesterol-containing atheromatous plaques and deposition of platelets within the endothelium, which narrow the arteries.

Initially poor blood flow through the coronary arteries to the myocardium is apparent only on exertion when oxygen demand is high – this results in the patient experiencing angina pectoris, which is chest pain caused by poor coronary blood flow. When the coronary arteries become occluded by thrombosis, or indeed if an area of atheromatous plaque breaks away and blocks an artery, there is no blood flow to the myocardium and the patient suffers a myocardial infarction. Drugs used to treat angina aim to increase coronary blood flow by vasodilation or reduce the workload of the myocardium to prevent high oxygen demand.

Diuretics

Diuretics are drugs that increase water excretion by the kidney. In heart failure, they reduce peripheral oedema and therefore preload, and reduce the congestion of pulmonary oedema: thiazide and loop diuretics are used together with potassium-sparing diuretics. Their use can result in rapid improvement in breathlessness (Swedberg *et al.*, 2005). Thiazide diuretics are also used in treatment of hypertension. Diuretics are considered in more detail later in the chapter.

ACE inhibitors

Examples: captopril, enalapril, ramipril and perindopril

Angiotensin-converting enzyme (ACE) inhibitors are drugs that inhibit the activity of ACE. ACE converts a precursor hormone angiotensin-1 to its active form angiotensin-2. Angiotensin-2 is a potent vasoconstrictor in blood vessels of the heart and the systemic circulation. It promotes release of the steroid aldosterone from the adrenal cortex, which stimulates vasoconstriction. ACE inhibitors are used clinically for the following reasons:

- to reduce peripheral vasoconstriction and blood pressure in hypertension;
- to reduce preload by venous dilation and reduce systemic blood pressure, to improve cardiac output in heart failure;
- to reduce overgrowth (hypertrophy) of the ventricular muscle, an action mediated by angiotensin-2.

The first drug in common use, captopril, had a short duration of action and was administered three times per day. It also had a profound hypotensive effect after the first dose, and a period of in-patient observation was often required to see if the patients tolerated its use. Newer ACE inhibitors like enalapril, ramipril and perindopril are prodrugs without the profound first-dose hypotension and therefore the onset of action is longer. They are available in once- or twice-daily prescriptions. It is still advisable, however, to initiate therapy at a low dose and titrate the dose against blood pressure.

ACE inhibitors are also used in diabetic patients to slow the rate of development of diabetes-related renal failure.

Side effects of ACE inhibitors are common:

- Hypotension can occur (which can be avoided with dose titration).
- Renal impairment can occur and it is advisable to monitor renal function after commencing therapy. This is more common in elderly patients with pre-existing renal artery disease or chronic kidney disease.
- A dry cough occurs in 10% of patients (Greenstein, 2004).
- High blood potassium level (hyperkalaemia) can occur, especially in patients with pre-existing renal disease or taking potassium-sparing diuretics.
- Rash, headaches and diarrhoea can occur.

Angiotensin receptor blockers

Examples: losartan, candesartan, valsartan and irbesartan

Angiotensin receptor blockers (ARBs) inhibit the angiotensin-2 receptors on the blood vessel wall and block the vasoconstrictor actions of angiotensin-2, therefore the indications or use of ARBs is the same as for ACE inhibitors. The side-effect profile is said to be better than for ACE inhibitors, and the incidence of cough is much less (Reid *et al.*, 2006).

Digoxin (digitalis)

Digoxin is a cardiac glycoside derived from the foxglove plant (digitalis). It acts to decrease sodium transport out of myocardial cells by inhibiting a cellular ion pump: sodium–potassium ATPase. As a by-product, this results in accumulation of calcium ions within the myocardium, and positive inotropism. It also inhibits the vagus nerve and reduces its influence on the sinoatrial and AV nodes. It therefore has two major clinical uses in heart disease (Reid *et al.*, 2006):

- as a positive inotrope it is used to increase CO in heart failure;
- it decreases ventricular rate in atrial fibrillation or atrial flutter by decreasing conduction across the AV node.

Digoxin can be given orally or intravenously, and a loading dose is often given to achieve rapid onset of peak blood level. Digoxin toxicity is quite common because there is a small difference between the therapeutic blood level and the toxic level. Thus, blood levels should be monitored closely and health professionals should recognise the signs of digoxin toxicity, as they can appear insidiously and mimic other disease presentations:

- Nausea and vomiting occur due to CNS stimulation.
- Acute or sub-acute onset of confusion, especially in the elderly.
- Altered colour vision, particularly yellow.

Cardiac effects also occur and are generally more obvious. These effects are potentiated when the blood potassium level is low (hypokalaemia):

- Bradycardia (less than 60 beats per minute).
- Complete heart block and collapse.
- Ventricular ectopic beats.

β-blockers

Examples: atenolol, carvedilol, propanolol, bisoprolol and metoprolol

β-blockers antagonise the effects of the sympathetic nervous system (SNS) by inhibiting β-adrenoreceptors, which are distributed throughout the body. β-Adrenoreceptors respond to circulating SNS catecholamines such as adrenaline and noradrenaline, which are released in times of stress and prepare the body for 'fight or flight' situations. They are classified as follows:

- *β-1 Adrenoreceptors*: predominantly in the heart; activation causes increased heart rate and positive inotropism.
- *β-2 Adrenoreceptors*: predominantly in the bronchi of the lungs, peripheral blood vessels and skeletal muscle. Activation causes bronchodilation, increasing airflow to the lungs, and vasoconstriction, leading to diversion of blood flow to the heart and brain.

The indications for the use of β-blockers are as follows:

- In hypertension, β-blockers reduce CO, peripheral resistance and activation of the renin–angiotensin, thus inhibiting sodium and water retention.
- β-Blockers are used in heart failure to reduce inappropriate SNS activation.
- β-Blockers are used as anti-arrhythmic drugs by reducing transmission through the electrical conducting system at all stages. They are therefore used in supraventricular tachycardias, atrial fibrillation and atrial flutter to reduce heartrate and restore sinus rhythm.
- β-Blockers are used as a treatment for angina, to reduce demand for coronary blood flow.

The adverse effects of β-blockers are related to exaggerated effects on the heart and also to effects on β-adrenoreceptors in other tissues.

Effects on the heart:

- Bradycardia (<60 beats per minute).
- Cardiogenic shock – too much negative inotropy may lead to profound hypotension and acute left ventricular failure in the acute setting. β-Blockers are normally withdrawn from treatment of heart failure when the patient is acutely unwell.

Peripheral effects:

- Peripheral vasoconstriction causing fatigue, cold peripheries and Raynaud's phenomenon.
- CNS reduced blood flow, leading to fatigue and vivid dreams.

- Bronchospasm via β-2 receptors in susceptible individuals with asthma or chronic obstructive pulmonary disease (COPD).

Calcium channel blockers

The contractility of vascular smooth muscle is dependent on the activity of calcium ion channels in the cell walls. Calcium channel blockers prevent influx of calcium into the cell and therefore reduce the contractility of blood vessel smooth muscle. They cause vasodilation in cardiac and systemic vessels. The class of drug is important because the site of action is different for each class. There are three classes of calcium channel antagonist:

- *dihydropyridines*: nifedipine and amlodipine;
- *phenylalkylamines*: verapamil;
- *benzothiazipines*: diltiazem.

Nifedipine and amlodipine have predominant peripheral vasodilator properties and are therefore used for the treatment of hypertension. Verapamil and diltiazem also have cardiac effects and are used to reduce heart rate (negatively chronotropic). They are used to terminate supraventricular tachycardias, atrial fibrillation and atrial flutter, as well as in the treatment of hypertension. The short-acting calcium channel blockers diltiazem and verapamil are often used in the treatment of angina pectoris due to potent vasodilation of coronary arteries. Nifedipine is a second-line agent in that respect.

Side effects are common. The dihydropyridines predictably cause headache, flushing and ankle swelling secondary to vasodilation. The anti-arrhythmic drugs can also precipitate bradycardia, heart block and asystole. As calcium channel blockers are often used in combination treatment with other negatively inotropic drugs (for example, β-blockers), dihydropyridines are preferred where possible to prevent hypotension and heart failure.

Nicorandil

Nicorandil is a potassium channel activator that causes vasodilation in systemic and coronary blood arteries and veins by opening potassium channels in the vessel smooth muscle wall. It is used as a second-line agent in the treatment of angina, when patients remain symptomatic despite having already taken β-blockers, nitrates or calcium channel blockers. A headache caused by cerebral vasodilation is a side effect that can occur in up to 50% patients. Nausea, dizziness, palpitations and flushing can also occur.

Nitrates

Nitrates are direct vascular smooth muscle relaxants that act on systemic arteries and veins to mediate their effects. Nitrates work in angina pectoris because vasodilation reduces preload and therefore lowers the workload on the myocardium. Additionally, coronary arteries are vasodilated directly to increase coronary blood flow. Intravenous nitrates are used for rapid vasodilation in the treatment of myocardial infarction and pulmonary oedema. Reduction in preload reduces myocardial oxygen demand, which subsequently has an increased inotropic effect and reduces systemic blood pressure.

Examples:

- *short-acting*: glyceryl-trinitrate (GTN);
- *long-acting*: isosorbide dinitrate and isosorbide mononitrate.

GTN is available as an aerosol spray, sublingual tablets, dermal skin patches or intravenous infusion. The aerosol is sprayed under the tongue when angina attacks occur. The tablets are administered sublingually, as GTN is poorly absorbed form the gut. They are left in situ for 20–30 min and then removed. The skin patches release GTN slowly over 24 h, producing a longer-lasting effect. Intravenous GTN is given via a syringe pump and the dose can be titrated to the severity of chest pain or blood pressure. Isosorbide dinitrate is prepared as a long-acting oral drug that is better absorbed than GTN. It is broken down to isosorbide mononitrate in the liver and is used in the maintenance treatment of angina pectoris.

Side effects of nitrates are common and are due to vasodilation:

- Headache, which can be severe and limits treatment.
- Palpitations.
- Hypotension due to systemic vasodilation. Patients can sometimes experience syncopal episodes after taking GTN spray.

Anti-arrhythmic drugs

There are a variety of anti-arrhythmic drugs in clinical usage. The mechanisms and clinical indications are listed in Table 8.1.

MEDICATIONS ACTING ON THE KIDNEYS

Oedema describes the retention of fluid by accumulation of water and sodium. The most common diseases that cause oedema are chronic heart failure, chronic liver disease (cirrhosis) and nephrotic kidney disease. In heart failure, low CO stimulates the kidney to activate the hormonal renin–angiotensin–aldosterone system. Aldosterone is produced by the adrenal cortex and acts on the distal tubule of the kidney to retain sodium and water to attempt to preserve circulating blood volume. This eventually leads to tissue oedema. Low levels of circulating plasma protein in cirrhosis (under-production) and nephrotic disease (loss of protein via the kidney) cause water to leak out from the blood capillaries into the peripheral tissues.

Patients who have oedema benefit from diuretics. These are drugs that act on the nephron of the kidney to increase the excretion of water and sodium chloride (Neal, 2005). All diuretics have this effect, but each acts in a slightly different way on the kidney and is classified accordingly.

The simple classification of diuretic drugs is:

- loop diuretics;
- thiazide diuretics;
- potassium-sparing diuretics;
- carbonic anhydrase inhibitors;
- osmotic diuretics.

Loop diuretics

Examples: furosemide and bumetanide

Loop diuretics act on the loop of Henle within the nephron (see Figure 8.3) to prevent re-absorption of sodium back into the circulation from urine being collected at this site. They produce a powerful diuresis.

Loop diuretics are indicated for treatment of oedema in heart failure, nephrotic syndrome and cirrhosis. Furosemide is the most common in use and is given orally to reduce peripheral

Table 8.1 Common anti-arrhythmic drugs in clinical usage

	Mechanism of action	Clinical indication	Adverse effects
Amiodarone	Prolongs conduction in all cardiac tissue by prolonging the cardiac action potential	Supraventricular tachycardia Atrial fibrillation and atrial flutter Ventricular tachycardia Little negative inotropic action, so safe in heart failure	Lung fibrosis Provokes ventricular tachycardia (torsade de pontes) Hepatitis Hypo- or hyper-thyroidism Photosensitivity
Sotalol	A β-blocker, but also prolongs cardiac action potential	Supraventricular tachycardia Atrial fibrillation and atrial flutter	As for β-blockers Torsade de pointes
Adenosine	Stimulation of purinergic receptors at SA and AV node, causing delay in conduction	Supraventricular tachycardia	Transient complete heart block Flushing (vasodilation) and chest tightness Contraindicated in asthma
Lidocaine	Slowing of conduction in Purkinje fibres and ventricular muscle	Ventricular tachycardia	Hypotension Bradycardia Nausea and vomiting
Flecainide	Slows conduction in atria, Purkinje fibres and ventricles	Atrial arrhythmias Supraventricular tachycardia	Ventricular arrhythmia and asystole Ataxia Taste disturbance

oedema, usually in a small daily dose. The dose is often increased and given intravenously for pulmonary oedema and severe peripheral oedema. Bumetanide is an alternative that is more readily absorbed from the gut than furosemide, when oedema is severe enough to affect the bowel wall.

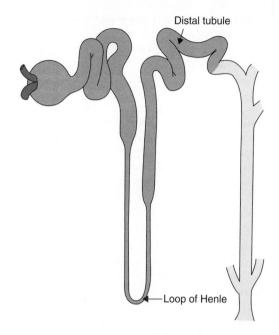

Fig 8.3 Parts of a nephron showing the site of action of loop diuretics (loop of Henle) and thiazides (distal tubule)

Side effects of loop diuretics are low blood potassium (hypo-kalaemia) from increased renal excretion, excessive salt and water depletion causing hypovolaemia, and low blood sodium (hyponatraemia). It is therefore important to monitor plasma urea, creatinine and electrolytes in patients on high doses of loop diuretic. Deafness and vertigo (ototoxicity) can result from large doses of furosemide. This is usually reversible on stopping the drug.

Thiazide diuretics

Examples: bendroflumethiazide (bendrofluazide), indapamide and metolazone

Thiazides act on the distal convoluted tubule to reduce the re-absorption of sodium by inhibiting a sodium and chloride ion pump. Water tends to follow sodium and they pass through the distal tubule and are excreted in the urine. The effect is slower and less powerful than that of loop diuretics. Thiazides also have a mild vasodilatory effect, particularly bendrofluazide. For this reason, they are also used in small doses for their anti-hypertensive effect.

Thiazides are indicated for treatment of heart failure, cirrhosis and nephrotic syndrome. In chronic heart failure metolazone is added to a loop diuretic, when the diuretic effect of the loop diuretic alone is not sufficient. Bendrofluazide is often used as a combination drug in the treatment of hypertension. In stroke disease in the elderly, the thiazide indapamide is used in combination with an ACE inhibitor to treat hypertension and reduce risk of further stroke.

Side effects of thiazide diuretics are:

- *Hypokalaemia* caused by increased excretion in the collecting ducts. This requires frequent measurement of serum electrolytes and potassium supplements. The risk is higher than for loop diuretics because thiazides have a longer duration of action.
- *Hyperuricaemia (gout)* occurs uncommonly and is caused by increased uric acid secretion.
- *Glucose intolerance and hyperlipidaemia* that are gradually progressive over months.
- *Impotence* is reported in 10% of middle-aged males using thiazides as anti-hypertensives (Waller *et al.*, 2001).

Potassium-sparing diuretics

Examples: spironolactone and amiloride

Potassium-sparing diuretics cause sodium and water loss without the unwanted effect of potassium excretion. Aldosterone is produced by the adrenal cortex in response to low CO and hypovolaemic circulation. It acts to retain sodium and water to increase circulating blood volume, at the expense of excreting potassium. Spironolactone is an aldosterone antagonist that prevents aldosterone binding to its cell receptor in the distal tubule, and therefore encourages sodium and water excretion and promotes potassium retention. Amiloride works in a slightly different manner and inhibits the action of aldosterone by competitively binding to its target sodium ion channels in the distal tubule. This causes sodium and water loss and also promotes potassium retention.

Potassium-sparing diuretics are indicated as oral preparations, on a once-daily basis for use in heart failure and cirrhosis. They are often used in combination with thiazides and loop diuretics to potentiate their effect and prevent potassium loss.

Unwanted effects are few but are a serious consideration. Hyperkalaemia can occur, which is more common in the presence of chronic kidney disease (which also causes hyperkalaemia) and in patients taking ACE inhibitors.

Hyponatraemia can occur in combination with other diuretics. Long-term use of spironolactone is avoided because gynaecomastia as a result of an oestrogenic effect and carcinogenic effect has been reported.

Carbonic anhydrase inhibitors

Example: acetazolamide

Acetazolamide antagonises sodium re-absorption in the proximal tubule and results in sodium and water loss, and by ion exchange also results in increased potassium excretion. However, it is rarely used as a diuretic as its effect is short lived. Its use is restricted to acute mountain sickness as a respiratory stimulant and in glaucoma to reduce intra-ocular pressure.

Its side effects are nausea, vomiting, dizziness, paraesthesiae and hypokalaemia.

Osmotic diuretics

Example: mannitol

Osmotic diuretics are simple compounds that are filtered at the glomerulus of the kidney and pass through the tubule without being re-absorbed into the circulation. They have an osmotic effect within the tubule that draws water along and prevents it from being re-absorbed. In that sense, they have no true pharmacological effect but just have an exaggerated physiological effect that results in excretion of water. The only osmotic diuretic in general use is mannitol, which is administered intravenously and has a short duration of action. Its most common use is for raised intracranial pressure after head injury, haemorrhage or neurosurgery. The osmotic effect reduces intracerebral oedema.

The main side effect is expansion of blood volume due to the osmotic effect. This can precipitate the onset of pulmonary oedema.

MEDICATIONS COMMONLY USED TO TREAT INFECTIONS

The introduction of the antibiotic to treat bacterial infection was one of the greatest medical advances of the twentieth century. There has been an increase in the number of agents used since the discovery of sulphonamides and penicillin, and now viruses and fungi are readily treated as well as bacteria. Reid *et al.* (2006) describe the issues that should be considered when choosing an appropriate antimicrobial agent for a patient. These are shown in Table 8.2.

Antimicrobial drugs can be classified according to the type of organism they target and the way they exert their pharmacological effect. This is not an exhaustive list, but all examples are in common usage.

- antibacterial drugs that inhibit DNA synthesis: sulphonamides, trimethoprim, quinolones, metronidazole and rifampicin;
- antibacterial drugs that inhibit cell wall synthesis: penicillins, cephalosporins and vancomycin;

Table 8.2 General principles of antimicrobial therapy

Patient factors	Organism factors	Drug factors
Document site of infection	Bacteria, virus or fungus	Absorption
Age	Typing	Tissue distribution
Renal and liver function	Culture and sensitivity	Route of elimination
General health and immune system		Adverse reactions
Pregnancy		

Adapted from Reid *et al.* (2006).

- antibacterial drugs that inhibit protein synthesis: aminoglycosides, tetracyclines and macrolides;
- antifungal drugs;
- antiviral drugs.

Antibiotics

One way of characterising antibacterial drugs (antibiotics) is to describe them as bacteriocidal (those that kill bacteria) or bacteriostatic (those that inhibit the growth and function of bacteria). However, there is not always a distinction between the two – large doses of most bacteriostatic agents are also bactericidal, whereas low concentrations of bacteriocidal agents are only bacteriostatic. Another way of defining antibiotics is by describing the type of bacteria that they are effective against. Gram staining (named after Danish scientist Hans Gram) 'colours' bacteria either violet (Gram positive) or red (Gram negative) when viewed under the microscope. Gram-negative bacteria have a different cell wall structure to Gram-positive bacteria and therefore have different antibiotic susceptibilities.

Sulphonamides

Sulphonamides (for example sulphamethoxazole) were the first group of drugs found to be effective, but they are little used as antibiotics now because of their low potency, microbial resistance and high incidence of adverse effects. Bacterial cells synthesise folic acid, which is vital for DNA synthesis, and sulphonamides inhibit an enzyme in susceptible bacteria, which prevents folic acid production. Although effective against a wide range of bacteria, the sulphonamides commonly cause rashes, renal failure, anaemia and bone marrow suppression. Trimethoprim is well absorbed orally and used effectively for treatment of simple cystitis. It is also used for respiratory tract infections on occasion but is not very effective against *Streptococcus pneumonia*, the bacteria most frequently implicated. Trimethoprim can cause harm to the foetus in the first three months of pregnancy (teratogenic) so should not be used. Co-trimoxazole, which is a combination of trimethoprim and sulphamethoxazole, is used for the treatment of *Pneumocystis jirovecii (carinii)* pneumonia, a common fungal infection in immunosuppressed patients.

Quinolones

Examples: ciprofloxacin, levofloxacin, norfloxacin and ofloxacin

The quinolones inhibit DNA-gyrase, an enzyme required for DNA synthesis in bacteria but not present in human eukaryotic cells. Ciprofloxacin acts against a wide range of bacteria, and is well absorbed orally and penetrates deep into tissue and cells (unlike penicillin). It is given twice a day orally or intravenously, but this gives no pharmacological advantage. Side effects include headache, rashes and diarrhoea, particularly *Clostridium difficile* infection. Reported outbreaks of infective diarrhoea have restricted its use to a second-line drug for urinary, abdominal and respiratory infection. However, it is the drug of choice for documented Gram-negative *Campylobacter jejuni*, *Salmonella* sp. and *Pseudomonas aeruginosa* infections. Quinolones raise blood levels of theophylline and warfarin therefore care should be taken with dosing of these drugs. Levofloxacin is more active against *Streptococcus pneumonia* than ciprofloxacin and is therefore used more in respiratory tract infection.

Metronidazole

Metronidazole damages or inhibits the synthesis of microbial DNA. It is active against anaerobic bacteria such as *C. difficile* and certain protozoal infections including *Entamoeba histolytica* (amoebic dysentery) and *Giardia lamblia* (giardiasis). Metronidazole is well absorbed orally but can be given intravenously. Side effects are rare, but prolonged use can cause peripheral neuropathy, and taking metronidazole with alcohol causes a chemical reaction between the two that leads to flushing, headache, vomiting and hypotension, so should be avoided.

Rifampicin

Rifampicin is effective against Gram-positive and Gram-negative bacteria, including methicillin-resistant *Staphylococcus aureus*, and also against *Mycobacterium tuberculosis* (TB). It inhibits RNA-polymerase, an enzyme in the microbial DNA synthesis pathway. It is well absorbed from the gut and is given orally in a once-daily dose. It is metabolised and excreted via the liver and can cause an elevation of liver enzymes, which is usually transient. However, care should be taken in patients with existing liver disease or alcohol problems. It can also interfere with the liver metabolism of other drugs such as warfarin, steroids and the oral contraceptive pill. Patients should be warned that their urine, tears and sputum will turn orange for the duration of treatment, and they should be monitored for renal impairment and low platelet count. In the treatment of TB, rifampicin is used in combination with isoniazid, ethambutol and pyrazinamide to prevent antimicrobial resistance developing.

Penicillins

Examples: benzylpenicillin, phenoxymethylpenicillin, flucloxacillin, ampicillin, amoxicillin and co-amoxiclav

All the penicillin antibiotics share a common structure, the β-lactam ring, which is a nitrogen-containing compound that prevents synthesis of the bacterial cell wall. However, many bacteria contain β-lactamase enzymes (penicillinase) that destroy penicillins, so the structure of penicillin has been modified a number of times to produce a whole family of penicillin antibiotics, with different bacterial susceptibilities.

Benzylpenicillin was the first penicillin to be used in clinical practice (Greenstein, 2004). It is given intramuscularly or intravenously and cannot be given orally. It has a narrow target range of bacteria and is limited to Gram-positive organisms such as *Staphylococcus* and *Streptococcus* (which often cause cellulitis, tonsillitis and pneumonia), and *Meningococcus* (which causes meningitis).

Phenoxymethylpenicillin is an alternative to benzylpenicillin with a similar antimicrobial range, which can be given orally. Flucloxacillin has a slightly different structure to benzylpenicillin, which means it can be used against some staphylococci that are resistant to benzylpenicillin. However, some staphylococci are resistant even to flucloxacillin, and these are called methicillin-resistant *Staphylococcus aureus*.

Ampicillin is an intravenous preparation that has a broad spectrum and is effective against Gram-negative organisms such as *Escherichia coli* and other Gram-positive organisms such as *Haemophilus influenzae, Listeria monocytogenes* and *Salmonella* spp.

Amoxicillin is better absorbed than ampicillin and can be given orally, and therefore is used more commonly for respiratory tract and urinary infections. However, resistance to both broad-spectrum drugs is common (>50% of staphylococcal infections, most *P. aeruginosa*, and 50% *E. coli* infections; Neal, 2005), so adding clavulanic acid to amoxicillin (co-amoxiclav) often results in a better outcome.

Penicillin resistance is common because many organisms that were originally sensitive to penicillin now produce penicillinase, which destroys the β-lactam ring. Several attempts have been made to produce β-lactam drugs that are resistant to penicillinase, namely cephalosporins, carbapenems and vancomycin. These are described below. The side effects of penicillins are few, but allergy is common and may present as rashes or even anaphylaxis (in 10% of allergies). Penicillins are excreted via the kidney, so toxicity can occur in established renal failure.

Cephalosporins

Examples: cefalexin, ceflacor, cefotaxime, cefuroxime, ceftriaxone and ceftazidime

Cephalosporins are a large group of antibiotics that all contain a β-lactam ring. Although they are rarely used as first-line agents (since there are cheaper, oral alternatives), they all have a broad spectrum of effectiveness. Older cephalosporins have now been superseded by newer ones, which are generally resistant to bacterial penicillinase. Oral first- and second-generation cephalosporins, such as cefalexin and ceflacor, are still used for respiratory tract infections caused by *H. influenzae* and urinary tract infections.

Third-generation cephalosporins are usually given intravenously and have a markedly increased activity against Gram-negative bacteria over the penicillins and earlier cephalosporins. They are also very effective against *Neisseria gonorrhoeae* and *H. influenzae*. Cefuroxime, cefotaxime and ceftriaxone (which is long acting) are used for blind treatment of severe infections such as pneumonia, meningitis and septicaemia. Ceftazidime is particularly useful against *P. aeruginosa*.

Side effects of the cephalosporins include diarrhoea, nausea, vomiting, abdominal distension, headache and allergic rashes. Outbreaks of infective diarrhoea in hospitals have limited their use more recently for blind treatment and prevention of abdominal infection in surgical patients.

Aminoglycosides

Examples: gentamicin, amikacin, tobramycin and neomycin

The aminoglycosides inhibit the synthesis of bacterial protein by binding to ribosomes within the bacterial cell (Downie *et al.*, 2003). They act in a bacteriocidal manner, and the full mechanism is not completely understood. The aminoglycosides are effective against many Gram-negative and a few Gram-positive organisms.

Gentamicin is the most prevalent aminoglycoside and is used for the treatment of severe infection such as Gram-negative septicaemia, meningitis, acute pyelonephritis and Gram-negative endocarditis.

Amikacin is used if gentamicin resistance has been proven. Neomycin and gentamicin are used as local drops in the treatment of external ear and conjunctival infection. Tobramycin is used in the treatment of *P. aeruginosa* infections.

Aminoglycosides are poorly absorbed orally and so are given intravenously and have a very narrow optimal range of concentration in the blood (therapeutic range). Blood levels must be taken either before dosing (trough level) or 1 h after dosing (peak level) to enable the prescriber to adjust the dose. Aminoglycosides are excreted by the kidney. Side effects are related to high plasma levels or long treatment courses, which can cause vertigo and deafness (ototoxicty), and renal impairment (nephrotoxicity). Care must be taken and the dose reduced in elderly patients, those with established kidney disease or those already taking furosemide.

Tetracyclines

Examples: doxycycline, minocycline and tetracycline

Tetracycline drugs are bacteriostatic and inhibit protein synthesis by reducing ribosomal activity. Tetracyclines have a broad spectrum of activity against many Gram-positive and Gram-negative infections. Of the three similar structured and commonly used tetracyclines, minocycline and doxycycline are longer-acting preparations than tetracycline and are therefore given in once-daily doses.

The main use of tetracyclines is first-line treatment against *H. influenzae* causing respiratory infections. Other infections treated with tetracyclines are atypical pneumonias (Q-fever, Lyme disease and mycoplasma pneumonia), non-specific urethritis (*Chlamydia*) and cholera (*Vibrio cholerae*). Minocycline is also indicated for the treatment of acne vulgaris.

Tetracyclines have an affinity for developing bone and teeth, which become discoloured brown, so it should be avoided in breastfeeding and pregnant women, and in young children. Mild gastrointestinal side effects are common such as nausea, vomiting and epigastric discomfort, but infective diarrhoea is rare.

Macrolides

Examples: erythromycin, clarithromycin and azithromycin

Macrolides are bacteriostatic antibiotics that act against the bacterial cell ribosome to prevent protein synthesis. Against some organisms they are bacteriocidal. Erythromycin has a spectrum of action that is similar to benzylpenicillin and is often used in its place in patients with penicillin allergy. Erythromycin is used for common and atypical respiratory tract and soft tissue infections. It can be given orally or by intravenous injection.

Clarithromycin and azithromycin are closely related to erythromycin and their uses are similar. It is thought that clarithromycin and azithromycin are more effective against *H. influenzae*, *H. pylori* (causing gastric ulcers) and organisms causing non-specific urethritis.

Side effects of macrolides are generally mild, and the drugs are tolerated well. Nausea, vomiting and diarrhoea can occur and are dose related. When erythromycin is given intravenously, it can cause irritation and thrombophlebitis, therefore for this route clarithromycin is often preferred.

Antifungal drugs

Two types of fungal infection exist (Downie *et al.*, 2003):

- topical infections (skin and mucous membranes);
- systemic infection.

Most fungal infection is opportunistic. The fungi involved live on the skin and mucous membranes but only cause infection when the patient is immunocompromised, for example on steroids or disease modifying anti-rheumatic drugs (DMARDs), or if local damp conditions permit fungal proliferation (for example, vaginal thrush in an obese patient).

Topical infections are common and commonly include athlete's foot (tinea pedis), ringworm (tinea corporis) or mucosal candidiasis (thrush). Drugs commonly applied locally or given orally to treat infection are imidazoles (ketoconazole and miconazole), which inhibit fungal cell enzymes, and triazoles (fluconazole) and polyenes (nystatin), which alter the permeability of cell membranes, resulting in loss of cell constituents. Nystatin is particularly effective against candidiasis. Other drugs such as griseofulvin and terbinafine are sometimes used.

Systemic fungal infection is usually treated with the polyene amphotericin, which is given intravenously, oral or intravenous triazoles, or intravenous imidazoles. Intravenous flucytosine is also used on occasion.

Topical therapy is virtually free of side effects, but amphotericin therapy is commonly associated with fever and rigors during the first week of therapy, nausea, vomiting and subsequently nephrotoxicity, which is dose related and limits its use.

Antiviral drugs

Viruses are smaller than bacteria and do not contain any enzymes that can be modulated. This is why antibiotics are not effective against viruses. A virus is essentially a core of nucleic acid protein (either RNA or DNA) and causes damage by replicating inside human (the host) cells and damaging cellular mechanisms.

Patients with intact immune systems can usually resolve viral infection fairly easily, and most viruses cause problems in patients who are immunosuppressed. Antiviral therapy is limited to a small number of drugs. Acyclovir inhibits viral DNA polymerase, an enzyme responsible for viral growth and replication. It is used orally for patients with varicella and herpes zoster infection (chicken pox and shingles) and genital herpes. Systemic and serious infections with varicella and herpes zoster (including acute encephalitis) are treated with intravenous acyclovir.

Famciclovir and valaciclovir are similar alternatives. These drugs are well tolerated but headaches, nausea and vomiting can occur.

Anti-HIV therapy has expanded rapidly in the last 20 years, and a number of antiviral drugs exist that prevent replication of HIV. Two main categories are reverse transcriptase inhibitors and protease inhibitors. They are usually used in combination, and further discussion is beyond the scope of this book.

MEDICATIONS COMMONLY USED TO TREAT PAIN AND INFLAMMATION

Pain is described as the subjective sensation of a painful (nociceptive) stimulus. A nociceptive stimulus is one that causes tissue damage and initiates a nervous system response. The response is relayed via the spinal cord to the cerebral cortex where the brain interprets the stimulus as pain. If the nervous impulses are interrupted the patient will not feel any pain. For example, a bed-bound patient developing a pressure sore on the heel would normally feel pain, as a physiological prompt to move the foot to prevent worsening. A paraplegic patient with transection of the spinal cord would not interpret the same stimulus as painful and would therefore not be prompted to move the foot. More care is therefore needed to protect these patients from developing pressure sores. Pain can arise from somatic structures, such as the skin, or from visceral internal organs. Somatic pain is typically sharp, burning, stabbing, gnawing or throbbing, whereas visceral pain is typically cramp-like or colicky. The response of an individual to pain is also influenced by psychological factors. This determines whether or not pain causes distress to the patient.

The neural pathways involved in pain sensation are complex and not entirely understood, but the most popular theory is 'gating' (Greenstein, 2004). The brain is subject to a constant input of low-intensity sensations (for example light touch, vibration from the skin). These travel from the periphery to the dorsal column of the spinal cord. From here they are relayed to the cerebral cortex.

High-intensity stimulation (for example application of a needle to the skin) activates peripheral nerves that terminate in a different place in the spinal cord. These 'open the gate' and are relayed to the cortex via the spinothalamic tract and the thalamus, instead of the low-intensity signals, where they are interpreted as pain. Additionally, 'descending impulses' from the brain act on the spinal cord to dampen transmission through the 'gate'. Drugs that relieve pain (analgesics) act at various sites along the pathways and include the following:

* *anti-inflammatories*: act locally at the damaged site to reduce the painful stimuli produced;
* *simple analgesia*: paracetamol, which acts on the CNS to reduce the action of mediators of pain;
* *opioid analgesics*: act on the brain and spinal cord to reduce sensation of pain.

Non-steroidal anti-inflammatory drugs

Acute inflammation describes the body's response to attack by pathogens such as bacteria and viruses, and also foreign body material, such as wood splinters or animal bites. There are two types of immune response: a local (innate) response at the site of injury and an acquired immune response involving activation of specific immune cells, such as T-cells and antibody producing B-cells (Greenstein, 2004).

Steroids act to dampen the acquired immune response and are considered later in this chapter. Non-steroidal anti-inflammatory drugs (NSAIDs) target the innate immune response. This response involves the activation of the pain-producing chemicals prostaglandin and bradykinin. At first, pain is a useful physiological stimulus to warn of a local attack on the immune system and prepare the patient to fight it. However, if pain is severe or ongoing it can be disabling. There are two cyclo-oxygenase (COX) enzymes that enable formation of prostaglandin, and these are called COX-1 and COX-2 (Greenstein, 2004). Prostaglandins produced by COX-2 cause pain and inflammation, whereas prostaglandins produced by COX-1 have a housekeeping role and enable a variety of the body's tissues to remain intact and function, for example the stomach mucosa.

NSAIDs have three desirable actions, which all result from the inhibition of COX-2 (Rang *et al.*, 2007):

- an anti-inflammatory action by decrease in the production of prostacyclin (a vasodilator prostaglandin) and less oedema and swelling;
- an analgesic effect by desensitisation of local nerve endings to bradykinin;
- an anti-pyretic effect (lower temperature) by inhibiting the prostaglandins that act on the hypothalamus in the brain to produce high fevers.

NSAIDs include:

- non-selective NSAIDs;
- salicylates (aspirin).

Examples of non-selective NSAIDs are ibuprofen, naproxen, diclofenac, indometacin, mefenamic acid and etodolac. Ibuprofen is usually the drug of first choice, with the lowest incidence of side effects, and is available over the counter. There is a considerable variation in patients' response to NSAIDs. Some of the NSAIDs, including ibuprofen, are available over the counter as gels or sprays for application on muscular pain and inflammation. Diclofenac is available as an intramuscular injection or suppository. Clinical uses of NSAIDs include:

- analgesia in painful conditions such as back pain, dysmenorrhoea and headache;
- anti-pyretic in infection, although paracetamol is usually preferred, because it lacks the gastrointestinal side effects;
- anti-inflammatory action in acute inflammation (for example in soft tissue injury) and in chronic inflammation (for example joint pain in rheumatoid arthritis).

Side effects of NSAIDs are common. Gastrointestinal disturbances such as dyspepsia (indigestion), gastric bleeding and peptic ulceration occur as a result of the inhibition of COX-1. Prostaglandins are also involved with maintenance of renal blood flow, thus prolonged use of NSAIDs can also cause renal failure, salt and potassium retention and hypertension. Allergy reactions occur and can present as an urticarial rash, hayfever or asthma.

Aspirin (acetyl-salicylic acid) was one of the earliest NSAIDs synthesised and has a variety of additional effects (for example as an anti-platelet agent in cardiovascular disease). Its indications as an anti-inflammatory are the same as the other NSAIDs. It is given as a tablet and absorbed rapidly in the gut, and its clinical effect lasts for up to 4 h.

In addition to the side effects mentioned, aspirin is linked with encephalitis in children (Reye syndrome), so its use should be restricted to adults. With large doses 'salicysm' can occur (Rang *et al.*, 2007), which is a syndrome consisting of dizziness, deafness and tinnitus with respiratory alkalosis. Additionally, in toxic doses from self- or accidental poisoning, a metabolic acidosis and renal impairment can occur. Care should be taken while giving aspirin with other drugs that can cause bleeding, such as warfarin.

Paracetamol

Paracetamol is a simple analgesic without any anti-inflammatory action. Paracetamol is thought to block the activity of hydroperoxides. Hydroperoxides are a by-product of the metabolism of arachidonic acid by COX. They exert a positive feedback on COX to increase its activity even further. Paracetamol acts to block this in the nervous system but does not reduce inflammation at the peripheral site.

Paracetamol is given orally and is well absorbed in the gut, and the onset of action peaks at 30–60 min. The effect lasts 2–4 h. With therapeutic doses, side effects are uncommon, but with large doses damage to the liver (hepatotoxicity) and kidneys can occur. Paracetamol is metabolised in the liver and in high doses the enzymes that act to cause its breakdown become quickly saturated. The remaining paracetamol is metabolised abnormally and causes damage to liver cells (hepatocytes). If patients are seen quickly enough after overdose, they can be given *N*-acetyl cysteine intravenously, which encourages paracetamol metabolism in the liver.

Opioid analgesics

Opiate receptors are located within the spinal cord and brainstem, and activation of these receptors modifies the signal of pain sensation from incoming neurons. Natural (endogenous) opioids such as the enkephalins, endorphins and dynorphins are released locally to act on these receptors and reduce the pain signal, causing analgesia. The most important receptor is called the μ (mu) receptor and is responsible for most of the therapeutic and unwanted effects within the CNS.

Opioid analgesics are synthetic substances that mimic endogenous opioids by causing a prolonged activation of opiate receptors, thus promoting analgesia.

Opioids can be classified as:

- *weak opioids*: codeine and dihydrocodeine;
- *strong opioids*: morphine, diamorphine (heroin), methadone, pethidine and fentanyl;
- *partial opioid agonists*: buprenorphine and tramadol.

Codeine and dihydrocodeine, which are similar, are given orally or intramuscularly and are broken down in the liver into morphine, which is responsible for the analgesic effect. Codeine itself has a low affinity for opiate receptors, but any larger doses promote side effects. Weak opioids are therefore used in mild-to-moderate pain only. Codeine is also used to suppress coughing and treat diarrhoea. It is often given in combination with paracetamol (for example as co-codamol) or with NSAIDs. Like strong opioids, codeine is subject to abuse and can cause dependence.

Strong opioids relieve all types of pain by depressing the CNS's appreciation of pain and by causing a euphoric effect, where the emotional effect of pain is dulled. Morphine and diamorphine (which is a modified version of morphine) are both potent analgesics. The only difference between them is that diamorphine may have a slightly quicker onset of action (Greenstein, 2004). Morphine can be given orally as morphine sulphate tablets (MST), which may be short acting and required up to six times a day, or slow release given twice a day, or as a solution. Morphine and diamorphine may be injected subcutaneously, intramuscularly or intravenously. Given intravenously, the analgesic effect is rapid and can last for 4h, depending on the severity of the pain. Given subcutaneously the onset of analgesia is slower.

After surgery or in terminal illness morphine or diamorphine can be given as a continuous intravenous or subcutaneous infusion, or via a patient-controlled analgesia pump. In myocardial infarction or pulmonary oedema, morphine or diamorphine is given to produce analgesia, allay anxiety and slow breathing rate and also to vasodilate the coronary arteries to allow better cardiac perfusion. Morphine is metabolised in the liver and excreted via the kidney. Opioids should therefore be used with caution in renal failure, as repeated dosing causes accumulation of the drug. Methadone is used orally as a long-acting substitute for morphine in the treatment of inhaled or injected opioid dependence and prevents opioid withdrawal. Pethidine is a short-acting, rapid-onset synthetic opioid that is used for biliary and ureteric colic predominantly because it does not cause smooth muscle contraction. Fentanyl is a short-acting, rapid-onset opioid given intravenously, transdermally or inhaled, and used for its sedative effect in anaesthesia.

Partial agonists at opiate receptors are strong analgesics but are potentially less addictive and lack the same side-effect profile. Buprenorphine is a partial agonist of the μ receptor and is usually given by injection or sublingual tablet. It is not as potent when given orally. Tramadol is a μ receptor partial agonist and also activates mono-aminergic (5-HT and noradrenaline) neurones that are responsible for dampening pain in the spinal cord. Tramadol can be given orally or by injection, but does cause significant nausea and vomiting.

Side effects of opioids are:

- respiratory depression and apnoea (stopping breathing);
- sedation, confusion or hallucination;
- hypotension and bradycardia;
- nausea and vomiting;
- constipation;
- pupillary constriction;
- urticarial rash and itching;
- tolerance and dependence.

Note that continuous treatment with opioids results in tolerance of the drug, and therefore larger and larger doses are required to have the same effect. In terminally ill patients, however, increasing pain often requires larger doses of opioids and does not necessarily reflect tolerance. In this context, dependence is also unimportant and, while the patient is in pain, dependence is unlikely to occur.

Corticosteroids (steroids)

Corticosteroids are used for the following reasons (Reid *et al.*, 2006):

- to suppress inflammation;
- as immune suppressants;
- as replacement therapy.

They are hormones usually synthesised by the adrenal cortex and have a range of physiological functions. The body's own (endogenous) steroids can be divided by their actions into two classes. These are described in Table 8.3.

For most therapeutic uses, synthetic glucocorticoids have replaced the more natural cortisol (hydrocortisone or cortisone) because they lack the salt- and water-retaining (mineralocorticoid) properties of cortisol, and therefore the potential side effects of electrolyte disturbance and hypertension. However, in the case of adrenal replacement therapy, hydrocortisone is given with a synthetic mineralocorticoid fludrocortisone to enhance both

Table 8.3 Physiological functions of steroids

Glucocorticoids	Mineralocorticoids
Cortisol (hydrocortisone)	*Aldosterone*
Reduce inflammatory response	Sodium and water retention
Reduce immune response	(via rennin–angiotensin)
Improve mood (euphoria)	Increased potassium excretion
Alter glucose and protein metabolism to increase glycogen deposition in the liver and increase circulating blood glucose	
Mobilise fat and redistribute to centripetal areas (weight gain)	
Increase in the number of red blood cells and platelets	
Reduced bone formation and increased calcium loss	
Significant mineralocorticoid activity	

gluco- and mineralocorticoid activity. Additionally, hydrocortisone is used orally and as an injectable preparation (intravenous or intramuscular) for replacement therapy and in the treatment of inflammation in septicaemic shock, anaphylaxis and acute severe asthma. It is also given as an injection for the treatment of acute adrenal insufficiency (Addisonian crisis, see below). Topical hydrocortisone preparations are used to treat inflammatory conditions of the skin such as eczema, and a variety of strengths can be prescribed.

Examples of synthetic glucocorticoids: prednisolone, methylprednisolone, dexamethasone and beclomethasone.

Synthetic glucocorticoids diffuse into cells and bind to the intracellular steroid receptor, which activates or inhibits protein synthesis to exert the characteristic physiological effects. Prednisolone is the most commonly used oral glucocorticoid, and its clinical uses include acute and maintenance treatment in the suppression of chronic inflammation in diseases such as rheumatoid arthritis and inflammatory bowel disease. It is also used for suppression of allergic inflammatory responses in the treatment of acute and chronic asthma. Suppression of the acquired immune system (mainly lymphocytes) is useful in patients with haematological malignancy such as leukaemia. Methylprednisolone is similar to prednisolone in potency and bioavailability and can be given as an injection for rapid suppression of inflammation. Dexamethasone is a very potent glucocorticoid, but with little mineralocorticoid action. This makes it useful for conditions such as cerebral oedema, where water retention would be a disadvantage (Neal, 2005). Beclomethasone is active topically and does not pass into the circulation very well. This makes it useful for the treatment of eczema as a skin preparation and of asthma via inhalation. There are a variety of other inhaled steroids available, for example budesonide and flixotide.

When inter-current illness occurs, such as a respiratory tract infection or diabetic crisis, patients taking steroids are warned that endogenous steroid production is low and more synthetic glucocorticoid is required. A patient who takes 10 mg prednisolone orally each day will require an increase in the dose, possibly to 20 mg daily until the illness has subsided.

Adverse effects of steroids are predictable because they are related to the physiological effects of the drug. They can be severe and are:

- weight gain and obesity;
- adrenal suppression of steroid production (also see Addisonian crisis);
- high blood sodium level (hypernatraemia);
- low blood potassium level (hypokalaemia);
- hypertension due to sodium and water retention;
- diabetes due to increased glucose production;
- osteoporosis due to reduced bone formation;
- psychosis and behaviour change;
- peptic ulceration;
- increased susceptibility to infection;
- muscle weakness and wasting;
- slowed growth in children.

Withdrawal of steroid treatment suddenly should be avoided unless the treatment course is very short (a few days) because this can precipitate an acute physiological withdrawal (adrenal insufficiency) called Addisonian crisis. The patient may complain of acute abdominal pain and vomiting, and on examination blood pressure will be very low, requiring fluid replacement urgently, and biochemistry will show low blood sodium level (hyponatraemia) and high blood potassium level (hyperkalaemia). The main treatment required is intravenous hydrocortisone until the clinical situation improves.

CONCLUSION

This chapter has provided an overview of the basic pharmacology of common medications. Medications commonly used in cardiovascular disease have been discussed. Medications acting on the kidneys have been outlined. Medications commonly used to treat infections, pain and inflammation have been discussed.

REFERENCES

Downie G, Mackenzie J, Williams A (2003) *Pharmacology and Medicine Management for Nurses*, 3rd edn. Churchill Livingstone, Edinburgh.

Greenstein B (2004) *Trounce's Clinical Pharmacology for Nurses*, 17th edn. Churchill Livingstone, Edinburgh.

Neal MJ (2005) *Medical Pharmacology at a Glance*, 5th edn. Blackwell Publishing, Oxford.

Rang HP, Dale MM, Ritter JM, Moore PK (2007) *Pharmacology*, 6th edn. Churchill Livingstone, Edinburgh.

Reid JL, Rubin PC, Walters M (2006) *Lecture Notes on Clinical Pharmacology and Therapeutics*, 7th edn. Blackwell Publishing, Oxford.

Swedberg K, Cleland J, Drexler H, *et al.* (2005) Guidelines for the diagnosis and treatment of chronic heart failure: executive summary. *Eur Heart J* **26**(11): 1115–1140.

Waller DG, Renwick AG, Hillier K (2001) *Medical Pharmacology and Therapeutics*. WB Saunders, Edinburgh.

FURTHER READING

Beckett NS, Peters R, Fletcher AE, *et al.* (2008) Treatment of hypertension in patients 80 years of age or older. *N Engl J Med* **358**: 1887–1898.

Clayton B, Stock Y, Harroun R (2006) *Basic Pharmacology for Nurses*, 14th edn. Elsevier, Philadelphia.

Gold HS, Moellering RC (1996) Antimicrobial drug resistance. *N Engl J Med* **335**: 1445–1453.

Grahame-Smith DG, Aronson JK (2002) *Oxford Textbook of Clinical Pharmacology and Drug Therapy*, 3rd edn. Oxford University Press, Oxford.

Hopkins SJ (1999) *Drugs and Pharmacology for Nurses*, 13th edn. Churchill Livingstone, Edinburgh.

Jordan S, Torrance C (1998) Hypertension. *Nurs Times* **94**: 50.

National Institute for Clinical Excellence (NICE) (2006) *The Management of Atrial Fibrillation*. NICE, London. Quick Reference Guide. Available at www.nice.org.uk/nicemedia/pdf/CG036quickrefguide.pdf [accessed on 4 November 2009].

National Institute for Clinical Excellence (NICE) (2006) *The Management of Hypertension in Primary Care*. NICE, London. Available at www.nice.org.uk/nicemedia/pdf/CG034NICEguideline.pdf [accessed on 4 November 2009].

National Institute for Clinical Excellence (NICE) (2008) *Chronic Kidney Disease*. NICE, London. Available at www.nice.org.uk/nicemedia/pdf/CG073NICEGuideline.pdf [accessed on 4 November 2009].

Shulman R, Davies R, Landowski R (2002) Drugs used in heart disease. *Nurs Times* **98**: 43.

Wood S (2002) Pain. *Nurs Times* **98**: 41.

9 | Administration of Oral Medication

Brian Gammon and Dan Higgins

INTRODUCTION

Errors of medicine administration are a growing problem in the health systems of many developed countries (Karnon *et al.*, 2009). Within the UK, the majority of medication errors are made by staff nurses (Smith, 2004). Given this and the fact that junior nurses are often thrust into the immediacy of oral medicine administration in a pressured environment, extreme caution is required by more junior staff when administering oral medication. The principles of medicine safety are discussed more fully in Chapters 6 and 7.

The aim of this chapter is to provide an overview of administration of oral medication.

LEARNING OUTCOMES

At the end of this chapter, the reader will be able to:

❏ Explore 'professional disposition' and administration of oral medication.
❏ Discuss the oral route for administration of medications.
❏ Describe the pharmacokinetics of oral medications.
❏ Discuss the pharmacodynamics of oral medications.
❏ Describe a suggested procedure for administering a medication orally.
❏ Discuss medication discharge information.

PROFESSIONAL PREDISPOSITION AND ADMINISTRATION OF ORAL MEDICATION

When administering any medicine, including oral medication, nurses are bound by both statute (law) and the stipulations of the professional body to which, as practitioners, they are accountable. The Nursing & Midwifery Council [Nursing & Midwifery Council (NMC), 2008] stipulates that nurses must provide a high standard of practice and care at all times. Nurses must also act within the legislation and professional responsibilities relating to medicines and must ensure that they are competent to administer medication.

Furthermore, any continuing professional development requirements must be addressed immediately. Nurses remain personally accountable for actions and omissions in practice and must always be able to justify those actions and omissions.

Preston (2004) notes that many nurses do not routinely reflect on the intricacies of medicine administration, only doing so when near misses or errors occur. Scott (2002) asserts that a previous lack of rigorous medicine management policies led to a degree of relaxation on the part of nurses. Nurses themselves identify constant interruptions and poor mathematical skills, heavy workload, new staff, solving other problems while administering medicines and advanced medicine preparation without rechecking as causes of error (Tang *et al.*, 2007).

The National Patient Safety Agency [National Patient Safety Agency (NPSA), 2003, 2004, 2007a] identified poor communication, complacency, failure to read notes, failure to follow protocols and miscalculation of doses as compounding factors in erroneous oral medicine administration. Lack of knowledge of therapeutic action has also been found to be a significant factor in medicine administration errors (Krähenbühl-Melcher *et al.*, 2007; Deans, 2005). Nurses must be aware of these factors and the accompanying danger of regarding medicine administration as merely a mechanistic task.

Also, continuing developments in the field of pharmacology mean that correspondingly more novel ways of medicine delivery will be formulated. It is therefore incumbent on nurses to maintain levels of competence by regularly updating of their knowledge through either formal educational initiatives or self-directed learning.

Nurses who administer oral medicines should be assessed for mathematical competence (Fry & Dacey, 2007) and also be educated concerning the potential problems that can arise from medication errors (Downie *et al.*, 2000), since poor knowledge of oral pharmaceutical agents has also been cited as a contributory factor in errors. Checks and error traps should be built into all medication processes (Smith, 2004), but the nurse cannot rely solely on the organisation of which they are a part to shield them from errors.

The proper professional disposition demands that nurses are active in seeking out methods to improve their own knowledge, thereby improving clinical practice and outcomes. The NMC (2008) states that patients must be able to trust nurses and trust in the efficacy of the care that nurses provide. As an example, Figure 1.1 illustrates the steps required for correct medicine administration. If any one of these steps is missed, harm could or will result.

THE ORAL ROUTE FOR MEDICATIONS

Administering medications via the oral route is the most common and easiest way, and there are many formulations for this purpose (Hopkins, 1999; Trounce, 2000). The oral route is acceptable to most patients and is relatively uncomplicated. The majority of patients are able to take oral formulations and expensive equipment is not required for delivery. Whilst administration of medicines orally is not free of potential complications and risks of adverse reaction exist, the oral route reduces certain possible risks to patients, notably those associated with intravenous access, pain from injections and an increased risk of infection transmission.

During the prescribing process the choice of route is influenced by many factors; if the gastrointestinal tract is functional and the specific therapeutic goals can be achieved with oral medication therapy, it should be considered in the first instance.

Types of oral medication

The types of medication that may be administered orally are given in Table 9.1. For the various indications of specific oral medicines the reader is referred to Chapter 8.

PHARMACOKINETICS OF ORAL MEDICATIONS

Pharmacokinetics can be defined as how medications move and are absorbed within the body. Smith and Aronson (2002)

Table 9.1 Formulations of oral medication

Tablets	Liquids, solutions and suspensions	Oral powders	Granules	Capsules	Oral sprays
Plain/regular tablets	Aqueous solutions	Bulk powders	Bulk granules	Modified-release capsules	Inhalers Sublingual sprays
Effervescent/water-soluble tablets	Elixirs	Divided powders	Divided granules	Plain/regular capsules	
Modified-release tablets	Linctuses	Powders for oral liquids			
Sublingual tablets	Suspensions				
Buccal tablets	Mouthwashes and gargles				
Coated tablets					
Lozenges (compressed tablets)					
Chewable tablets					
Orodispersible tablets					

Adapted from Thacker *et al.* (2008).

summarise four principal elements of pharmacokinetics: absorption, distribution, metabolism and excretion. These are important considerations when assessing the dose and likely therapeutic impact of a medicine (Hopkins, 1999). Fogueri and Singh (2009) note that medicines have a unique set of properties contingent on their chemical and physical makeup, which must be considered in the choice of therapeutic agent in order to maximise the bioavailability of the medicine (bioavailability being the amount of a substance that reaches target receptors to exert a chemical action).

Absorption

The process of absorption brings the medicine from the site of administration into the circulatory or lymphatic system. A disadvantage of oral agents is that, despite convenience and ease of administration, there is often decreased bioavailability (when compared to intravenously administered medicines, for example, where bioavailability is 100%). The degree of bioavailability is affected by the degree of physical and chemical instability in the presence of gastric enzymes and the effects of harsh acidic environments.

The potency of many types of oral medications is also negatively affected by first-pass metabolism. First-pass metabolism is the phenomenon whereby medicines may be significantly altered by the action of the liver in its role in metabolising any potential toxins that enter the body. Many medicines are therefore broken down into metabolites and excreted before they reach the systemic circulation and can exert their therapeutic effects. Second- and third-pass metabolisms can occur in the stomach and the small intestine (the latter site is where the vast majority of drug absorption occurs). Other factors that affect oral medicine metabolism are given in Table 9.2.

Most medicines are absorbed via the gastrointestinal tract, which is why the oral route is the most common, but again a number of factors may positively or negatively influence the absorption of a medicine from the gut (Hopkins, 1999). These include gut motility, gastric emptying, surface area, gut pH, blood flow, presence of food and fluid in the gastrointestinal tract, concomitant therapy such as antacids and medicine composition [Royal College of Nursing (RCN), 2009].

Table 9.2 Factors influencing medicine metabolism

Age	The very young (detoxification systems not developed) and older people (reduced glomerular filtration rate and increased renal insufficiency) may not metabolise and excrete medicines very effectively
Bodyweight	The larger the person, the larger the area available for medicine distribution – size may affect the dosage required
	All patients should have their weight measured and recorded at regular intervals.
Pregnancy and lactation	Some medicines can cross the placenta or be transferred to the baby via breast milk
	Some medicines are capable of causing foetal abnormalities
Nutritional status	Malnourishment – particularly protein, fat and fluid deficits – alter the metabolism and availability of medicines
	A nutritional assessment of patients is therefore essential
Food–medicine interactions	Some foods can enhance or inhibit a medicine being absorbed, i.e. grapefruit juice potentiates the action of statins
Disease processes	Circulatory, liver and kidney diseases can reduce the distribution, metabolism and excretion of medicines, respectively
	In hepatic disease, larger amounts of the medicine may escape first-pass metabolism
Mental and emotional factors	If a patient is confused, is forgetful or has particular beliefs about a medicine, their ability to take it as recommended will be affected, as will overall compliance. There is a danger therefore that disease processes and symptoms will be unabated or will re-emerge
Genetic and ethnic factors	Medicine metabolism is partly determined by genetic makeup and its effect on the action of specific enzymes, e.g. the incidence of statin-induced myopathy is due to the presence of a genetic polymorphism
Polypharmacy	Many medicines have the capacity to potentiate or inhibit the effects of other medicines, e.g. simvastatin is known to increase circulating plasma levels of warfarin whilst iron preparations and tetracycline should be administered separately, as simultaneous administration will decrease the absorption of both (Downie *et al.*, 2000)

Adapted from RCN (2009); additional comments by Downie *et al.* (2000).

Distribution

Distribution involves the transportation of the medicine to the target site. Factors influencing distribution include blood flow and cardiac output, plasma protein binding, lipid solubility (highly lipid soluble medicines will readily cross the cell membrane), the placental barrier, blood–brain barrier and storage sites (RCN, 2009).

Metabolism

Medicine metabolism refers to modification of the chemical composition of the medicine. The pharmacological activity of the medicine is normally removed and metabolites produced. The main site of medicine metabolism is the liver, but metabolism may also occur in the kidneys, intestinal mucosa, lungs, plasma and placenta. Repeated use of some medicines may result in medicine tolerance, i.e. greater doses of the medication will be required to produce the same therapeutic effect.

Medicine interactions should also be considered; some medicine dosages may need to be adjusted to compensate for the enzymatic secondary effects of other medications taken simultaneously.

Excretion

Medicines are excreted through the following routes: saliva, sweat and tears, lungs, bile, kidneys, and the gastrointestinal tract. The processes of medicine metabolism and medicine excretion will ultimately determine the medicine's half-life. The half-life of a medicine is defined as the time required for plasma concentrations of a given medicine to decrease by 50% (Downie *et al.*, 2000). An effective plasma level of medicine may need to be reached quickly. This requires a loading dose of the medicine to be given. The maintenance dose then maintains a stable plasma level.

PHARMACODYNAMICS OF MEDICATIONS

Pharmacodynamics can be defined as the actions and effects of drugs. In order to exert their effect, medicines must reach cells via the processes of absorption and distribution already described.

Once at their site of action, medicines may work in a very specific manner or non-specifically. Specific factors include:

- interaction with receptors on the cell membrane;
- interference with ion passage through the cell membrane;
- enzyme inhibition or stimulation;
- interference with metabolic processes of microorganisms.

Non-specific factors include chemical alteration of the cellular environment and physical alteration of the cellular environment.

SUGGESTED PROCEDURE FOR ADMINISTERING A MEDICATION ORALLY

Preparation of oral medication and equipment

- Ensure that local policies and guidelines regarding the administration of oral medicines are followed (Smith, 2004).
- If a ward-based trolley system is used, check that all equipment that may be needed during the medicine round is present before commencing medicine administration.
- Where appropriate, ensure that mixtures are prepared sufficiently in advance following the instructions given on the pack insert. Local policies may differ for certain medicines in particular specialities; these should be agreed with the pharmacist.
- Check that the most commonly used medicines, i.e. those medicines that have a high probability of being required during the medicine round, are available in sufficient quantity to avoid leaving the trolley to restock.
- Follow local infection control guidance. Downie *et al.* (2000) note that prior to administration of any medicine the hands should be socially clean.
- Ensure that medicine administration rounds are integrated into ward routine to optimise correct frequency. Timing of medication administration is important. Studies have demonstrated administration-time-dependent effects on the therapeutic outcome (Zhu *et al.*, 2008).

- Ensure that sufficient time is available to undertake medicine-related tasks to a sufficiently high standard. 'Protected' medicine rounds have been suggested (Fry & Dacey, 2007). These minimise the impact of interruptions by other members of the multidisciplinary team, patients and relatives or phone calls.

Patient assessment

- Ensure that baseline assessment has been undertaken; this is highly important in preventing hypersensitivity reactions (Viale, 2009).
- Instances of adverse medicine reactions relating to polypharmacy and medicine interaction, particularly in the elderly, are an increasing phenomenon (O'Mahony & Gallagher, 2008). For this reason, it is important to determine the actual clinical need of a medication. Although nurses are reported to spend approximately 40% of their time in medicine administration, Downie *et al.* (2000) assert that the nurses' aim should be to reduce the need for medication.
- How old is the recipient? Depending on the age of the patient, an adjustment of the prescribed dose may be necessary, for example elderly patients tend to have reduced renal function despite having a normal creatinine level due their reduced muscle mass. In such instances, dose adjustments may be recommended and are usually proposed by the pharmacist.
- Time must be taken to provide explanations of the possible risks and benefits of the prescribed therapy to the patient in order to ensure their compliance. The NMC recommends that treatment plans involving medication are undertaken wherever possible, with the full informed consent of the person receiving the medicines. Patient education is also known to increase compliance both within hospital and once discharged (Moreira *et al.*, 2008; Peterson *et al.*, 2008). Wherever possible, therefore, the nurse should act as a facilitator of medication administration rather than an overseer.
- Do not use subterfuge in the administration of medicines. The NMC has produced guidelines concerning the disguising of medicines in food. 'As a general principle, by disguising medication in food or drink, the patient or client is being led to

believe they are not receiving medication, when in fact they are. The NMC would not consider this to be good practice'. (NMC, 2004).

- Know the therapeutic uses of the medicine to be administered, as well as normal dosage, side effects, precautions, interactions and contraindications.
- Ensure that the formulation of the medicine is appropriate to the patient.
- Be aware of the patient's plan of care. Unfamiliarity with patients is a significant source of medicine error (Nichols *et al.*, 2008).
- Assess the patient's likely compliance with the treatment regimen. Conditions such as diabetes significantly impair a person's ability to comply with oral medication plans.
- Cognitive assessment is vital. Assessment tools such as the Mini Mental State Examination (MMSE) are readily available and should form part of a person's initial admission assessment (Miura *et al.*, 2007). A simple internet search will provide the reader with large amounts of further information regarding the MMSE and other cognitive assessment tools.
- Patient weight is extremely important in calculating the dose of certain medications. This should be ascertained regularly and accurately, and be written on the prescription chart as well as the observation chart.
- Assess the probable effectiveness of the treatment prescribed. Are there factors that may limit the effectiveness of prescribed medicines? Some medicines, for example, react with nasogastric feeding tubes and are less potent as a result.
- Can the person swallow sufficiently well? Does their level of consciousness mean that the administration of oral medication may constitute a hazard? If a patient has a degree of dysphagia and you are using a syringe to give them medication orally, a speech and language therapist's input is strongly advised by the NPSA (2007b).

Implementation (administration) (Figure 9.1)

- Have medicines been stored correctly? Check the condition of the medication. Ensure that tablets are undamaged and

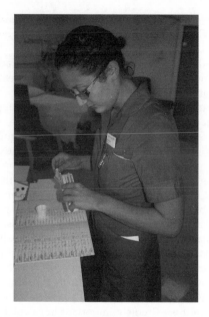

Fig 9.1 Administration of oral medication

suspensions are sufficiently mixed by inverting the container 8–10 times. If in doubt do not use but contact the pharmacist.
- Check the expiry date of the medication.
- Check the prescription thoroughly. In particular, the nurse must ensure that the prescription contains the following information (Downie *et al.*, 2000): the patient's name, address, hospital, ward, age, date of birth and unit number.
- The nurse should also check the date of prescription of each individual medicine, the full name of the medicine prescribed (using approved generic name), the dosage, the route or method of administration, the time of administration, and that a full signature of a registered prescriber is present.
- Ensure also that the medicine is due to be administered and has not already been given.
- The hands should not come into contact with the medicine unless this is unavoidable.

- Capsules and bottled tablets should be tipped out into the container lid before being transferred to the medicine beaker.
- Medication in blister packs should be pushed through the foil side of the pack.
- Tablets should not be crushed or broken (unless scored) but should be administered in the form in which they are prescribed. As Van den Bemt *et al.* (2006), crushing of tablets results in a higher initial blood level, increasing risk of adverse drug reactions (ADRs), a lower blood level nearer the end of the medicine action, increasing the potential for symptom recurrence, irritation of the gastric mucosa and a possible loss of effect.
- If a medicine is to be given via an enteral feeding-tube, specific advice from a pharmacist or nutrition specialist nurse should be sought. It is important to ensure that when delivering medications via this route the formulation is appropriate. It is not acceptable to assume that a medicine that can be given orally is appropriate for enteral tube administration.
- Check the identity of the patient using the required number of sources of information to establish identity beyond doubt. Between February 2006 and January 2007, the NPSA (2004, 2007a, 2008) received over 24 000 reports of patients and their care being mismatched, of which 2900 reports resulted from incidents concerning wristbands. From September 2009, the NHS identifier number must be used for all patient identification (NPSA, 2009).
- The nurse should remain by the patient's bedside to render any assistance necessary, to provide information where needed and to ensure that the medication has been taken correctly.
- The nurse should exercise discretion based on sound knowledge during the administration of oral medication and be aware of situations when it would be inadvisable to give medications. The withholding of digoxin if the person is experiencing bradycardia provides a common example.
- If the patient is 'nil by mouth' but has an intact swallowing reflex, the nurse must ensure that correct steps are followed. Many medications (notably anti-hypertensives) can be safely given with a small amount of water. Such medications form an important part of pre-operative or pre-investigation care

and should not simply be withheld (Corfield *et al.*, 2006), as abrupt withdrawal can provoke symptoms, depending on the type of medication involved. A doctor or pharmacist should be contacted for advice and, if necessary, alternative medications or routes should be used.

- If the medication is withheld for any reason, this should be documented on the prescription chart and in the nursing notes. It may be prudent in most cases to inform a clinician (NMC, 2008).
- The NPSA recommends that an appropriate oral/enteral syringe should be used to measure oral liquid medicine if a medicine spoon or graduated measure cannot be used. Oral/enteral syringes are colour coded purple and labelled 'oral/enteral' in bold type; they are sterile and single-use only (NPSA, 2007b).
- Intravenous syringes should not be used to measure and administer oral liquid medicines. Only well-labelled oral/enteral syringes that do not allow connection to an intravenous catheter or port should be used (NPSA, 2007b).
- Any enteral syringe with liquid medication in it that needs to be left unattended for any length of time must be labelled with the medicine name, dose, data and time of preparation, and nurses' signature (NPSA, 2007b).
- If the medicines' trolley must be left unattended, it should be locked and steps should be taken to ensure that it cannot be moved.
- Once the medicine has been administered, the nurse should date and initial the relevant parts of the prescription sheet.

Evaluation (after care)

- Take immediate steps to treat ADRs such as anaphylaxis.
- Contact the prescriber immediately if any ADRs are discovered.
- Make a clear, accurate and immediate record of all medication administered or withheld (NMC, 2008).
- Ensure patient comfort following the administration of the medicine. Inform them of any possible expected reactions and ensure that their dignity, health and safety are maintained.

Provide a means of summoning assistance. Provide other equipment that may be needed (e.g. commode) and place within easy reach.

- Monitor plasma concentrations of the medicine when requested to do so by the prescriber.
- Ensure that any changes to treatment plans are handed over accurately to nursing teams on subsequent shifts.
- Beakers and other equipment should be washed and dried after use according to local policy.

MEDICATION DISCHARGE EDUCATION

Medication discharge education (MDE) is especially important. Side effects are poorly understood by patients, and the risk of falls is significantly increased in the presence of certain classes of medication (McGraw & Drennan, 2001). Rycroft-Malone *et al.* (2000) assert that client education by nurses falls far short of expectations and consists mainly of information giving on the day of discharge (see also McGraw & Drennan, 2001). Both studies indicate that the best method of achieving optimum medication compliance, particularly among older persons, is by introducing adequate multidisciplinary assessment and a formalised education strategy rather than simply giving information.

Reiley *et al.* (1996) showed that nurses believed that 95% of patients understood the side effects of their medication but that only 57% of patients claimed that they understood. Reeson & Wafer (2001) found that of medication history obtained from 34 clients, 21 were taking at least three or more medications that were associated with increased risk of falls. A further four clients were known to have had falls directly related to medication. Medicine administration, particularly at discharge, should not be seen as an activity conducted in isolation. Reference should be made to other members of the multidisciplinary team where applicable. The involvement of pharmacists in particular has been shown to reduce the incidence of ADRs.

CONCLUSION

Medicine administration is a complex process. Nurses should be aware throughout this process of the consequences that accrue to any act or omission that could result in (sometimes severe) harm to a patient in their care. Nurses are responsible for the majority of mistakes involving medicines, but the antecedents to these mistakes are not necessarily the fault of nurses. Prescription errors and patient misidentification errors, for example, are common antecedents to errors of administration with the nurse as the last (often most telling) link in the chain. Nurses should therefore be aware of their position in this hierarchy and the possibility of compounding previous mistakes. The information within this chapter highlights the need for verification at every stage in the preparation, prescription and administration of oral medicines. Nurses must develop a mentality that is alert to the possibility of error and translated into evidence-based, responsive, systematic and consistent practice.

REFERENCES

Corfield LF, Trivedi PM, Wilson D (2006) Preoperative cardiac drug administration in general surgical patients: a completed audit. *Int J Clin Pract* **60**(10): 1300–1302. Epub 30 August 2006.

Deans C (2005). Medication errors and professional practice of registered nurses. *Collegian* **12**(1): 29–33.

Downie G, Mackenzie J, Williams A (2000) *Pharmacology and Medicine Management for Nurses*, 2nd edn. Churchill Livingstone, London.

Fogueri LR, Singh S (2009) Smart polymers for controlled delivery of proteins and peptides: a review of patents. *Recent Pat Med Deliv Formul* **3**(1): 40–48.

Fry MM, Dacey C (2007) Factors contributing to incidents in medicine administration: part 2. *Br J Nurs* **16**(11): 676–681.

Hopkins SJ (1999) *Medicines and Pharmacology for Nurses*, 13th edn. Churchill Livingstone, London. Available at www.npsa.nhs.uk [accessed on 4 November 2009].

Karnon J, Campbell F, Czoski-Murray C (2009) Model-based cost-effectiveness analysis of interventions aimed at preventing medication error at hospital admission (medicines reconciliation). *J Eval Clin Pract* **15**(2): 299–306.

Krähenbühl-Melcher A, Schlienger R, Lampert M, Haschke M, Drewe J, Krähenbühl S (2007). Medicine-related problems in hospitals: a review of the recent literature. *Med Saf* **30**(5): 379–407.

McGraw C, Drennan V (2001) Self-administration of medicine and older people. *Nurs Stand* **15**(18): 33–36.

Miura M, Kakei M, Iwasawa S, *et al.* (2007) Assessment of compliance for oral medicines with MMSE, Mini-Mental State Examination, in hospitalized elderly patients. *Yakugaku Zasshi* **127**(10): 1731–1738.

Moreira LB, Fernandes PF, Mota RS, *et al.* (2008) Medication noncompliance in chronic kidney disease. *J Nephrol* **21**(3): 354–362.

National Patient Safety Agency (NPSA) (2003) *Seven Steps to Patient Safety: a Guide for NHS Staff*. NPSA, London.

National Patient Safety Agency (NPSA) (2004) *Right Patient, Right Care: a Framework for Action – Final Report*. Available at www.npsa.nhs.uk/health/publications [accessed on 4 November 2009].

National Patient Safety Agency (NPSA) (2007a) *Safety in Doses: Improving the Use of Medicines in the NHS*. NPSA, London. Available at www.npsa.nhs.uk/healtj/publications [accessed on 4 November 2009].

National Patient Safety Agency (NPSA) (2007b) Bulletin 19: Promoting Safer Measurement and Administration of Liquid Medicines via Oral and Other Enteral Routes. NPSA, London.

National Patient Safety Agency (NPSA) (2008) *Safety in Doses: Medication Safety Incidents within the NHS* (4th report). NPSA, London.

National Patient Safety Agency (NPSA) (2009) *Risk to Patient Safety of Not Using the NHS Number as the National Identifier for All Patients*. NPSA, London.

Nichols P, Copeland TS, Craib IA, Hopkins P, Bruce DG (2008) Learning from error: identifying contributory causes of medication errors in an Australian hospital. *Med J Aust* **188**(5): 276–279.

Nursing and Midwifery Council (NMC) (2004) Guidelines for the administration of medicines. Available at www.nmc.org [accessed on 4 November 2009].

Nursing and Midwifery Council (NMC) (2008) Standards for medicines management. Available at www.nmc.org [accessed on 4 November 2009].

O'Mahony D, Gallagher PF (2008) Inappropriate prescribing in the older population: need for new criteria. *Age and Ageing* **37**: 138–141. Published by Oxford University Press on behalf of the British Geriatrics Society.

Peterson ED, Albert NM, Amin A, Patterson JH, Fonarow GC (2008) Implementing critical pathways and a multidisciplinary team approach to cardiovascular disease management. *Am J Cardiol* **102**(5A): 47G–56G.

Preston RM (2004) Medicine errors and patient safety: the need for a change in practice. *Br J Nurs* **13**(2): 72–78.

Reeson C, Wafer M (2001) Falls in accident and emergency departments. *Nurs Stand* **15**(50): 33–37.

Reiley P, Iezzoni LI, Phillips R, Davis RB, Tuchin LI, Calkins D (1996) Discharge planning: comparison of patients' and nurses' perceptions of patients following hospital discharge. *IMAGE: J Nurs Scholarship* **28**(2):143–148.

Royal College of Nursing (RCN) (2009) Available at www.rcn.org.uk [accessed on 4 November 2009].

Rycroft-Malone J, Latter S, Yerrell P, *et al.* (2000) Nursing and medication education. *Nurs Stand* **14**(50): 35–39.

Scott H (2002) Increasing number of patients are being given wrong medicines. *Br J Nurs* **11**(1): 4.

Smith DG, Aronson JK (2002) *The Oxford Textbook of Clinical Pharmacology and Drug Therapy*, 3rd edn. Oxford University Press, Oxford.

Smith J (2004) *Building a Safer NHS for Patients: Improving Medication Safety*. Department of Health, HMSO, London.

Tang FI, Sheu SJ, Yu S, Wei IL, Chen CH (2007) Nurses relate the contributing factors involved in medication errors. *J Clin Nurs* **16**(3): 447–457.

Thacker M, Samuel I, Atkinson H (2008) Oral medicine administration guidelines (for adults). *Hospital Guideline Document*. Royal Free Hampstead NHS Trust, London.

Trounce J (2000) *Clinical Pharmacology for Nurses*. Churchill Livingstone, Edinburgh.

van den Bemt PM, Cusell MB, Overbeeke PW, *et al.* (2006) Quality improvement of oral medication administration in patients with enteral feeding tubes. *Qual Saf Health Care* **15**(1): 44–47.

Viale PH (2009) Management of hypersensitivity reactions: a nursing perspective. *Oncology* (Williston Park) **23**(2 Suppl 1): 26–30.

Zhu LL, Zhou Q, Yan XF, Zeng S (2008) Optimal time to take once-daily oral medications in clinical practice. *Int J Clin Pract* **62**(10): 1560–1571.

Administration of Injections

10

Janet Hunter

INTRODUCTION

The administration of intradermal (ID), subcutaneous (SC) and intramuscular (IM) injections is a vital part of drug administration and in clinical practice is a common nursing intervention. These parenteral methods of administration are used to instil medications directly into the tissues. The procedures used are invasive and therefore present greater risks than alternative methods such as the oral and topical routes. When injected, they act more quickly as they are absorbed through the tissues. Hence, the effective and safe administration of medications via these routes is determined by performing a safe and competent technique, the clinical outcome and whether any adverse effects are experienced by the individual (Shepherd, 2002).

Medicines management is an important aspect of professional practice. When administering injections, the nurse is responsible for the administration of a range of prescribed medications using ID, SC and IM routes. To achieve this, the Standards for Medicines Management from the Nursing & Midwifery Council [Nursing & Midwifery Council (NMC), 2008] provide guidance so that nurses can perform safe and accountable practice. This requires the nurse to posses the knowledge and principles that underpin these skills as well as thought and the exercise of professional judgement.

The aim of this chapter is to provide an overview to the administration of injections. The administration of IV injections will be discussed in Chapter 11.

LEARNING OUTCOMES

At the end of this chapter, the reader will be able to:

❑ List the routes for administration of injections.
❑ Discuss the location and selection of the appropriate injection site.
❑ List the factors to consider when selecting an injection site.
❑ Discuss the complications associated with ID, SC and IM injections.
❑ Describe the principles of practice for administering injections.

ROUTES FOR ADMINISTRATION OF INJECTIONS

The choice of route is determined by the required pharmacological outcome, patient comfort and safety. Although the ID route is used mainly for allergy testing, there are other considerations when choosing the SC or IM injection route, for example:

• The medication needs to be absorbed relatively quickly, which is achieved when the drug is absorbed into the bloodstream rather than the gastrointestinal tract (Rodger & King, 2000).
• The medication will be altered or destroyed by the gastrointestinal tract, e.g. insulin.
• The individual is nil by mouth.
• A prolonged release of the drug is required for optimum therapeutic effect, e.g. depot injections.
• The drug is only manufactured as an injection, e.g. vaccines, heparin and insulin.

The three common parenteral routes for administering medications are discussed below.

Intradermal route

The ID route is chosen to provide a local, rather than a systemic, effect. It is primarily used for diagnostic purposes such as allergy or tuberculin testing, although it is also used when a local anaesthetic is needed prior to an invasive procedure (Workman, 1999; Corben, 2005). The medication is injected into the dermis just under the epidermis, where the blood supply is reduced. This is ideal as a prolonged absorption and action is required, and the medications tend to be potent.

Only small amounts of solution are injected, ranging from 0.1 to 0.5 ml, until a wheal appears on the skin surface (Workman, 1999; Perry & Potter, 2006). Importantly, sites must be labelled when testing for allergies so the antigen and response can be clearly identified. With allergy testing, treatment for anaphylactic shock needs to be accessible in case the individual experiences hypersensitivity or allergic reaction.

Subcutaneous route

The SC route for injections is recommended when a slow, continuous absorption of the drug is required, for example insulin and low-molecular heparin. This route is also relatively pain free. The medication is injected into the fat and connective tissue, below the dermis. There is less blood flow in the SC tissues and therefore the absorption rate is slower.

The amount of solution that can be given must not exceed 2 ml (Chan, 2001; Nicol *et al.*, 2008). Highly soluble medications are usually injected, which prevents irritation of the skin and tissues (Workman, 1999).

Intramuscular route

Injection via the IM route is chosen when a reasonably rapid systemic uptake of the drug is required, usually between 15 and 20 min, and a relatively prolonged action is needed. Medications given via this route include analgesics, anti-emetics, sedatives, immunisations, hormonal treatments and antibiotics. The amount of solution that can be injected depends on the muscle bed. For adults this ranges from 1 to 5 ml, although much smaller volumes are acceptable for children (Rodger & King, 2000; Watt, 2003; Greenway, 2004; Corben, 2005).

The medication is usually injected into the denser part of the muscle facia underlying the SC tissues. As skeletal muscle is less sensitive to potent and viscous drugs and can absorb higher volumes, this is ideal when a rapid uptake of the drug is required into the bloodstream via the muscle fibres. As there are also fewer pain-sensing nerve endings in muscle, when administered correctly, IM injections should be less painful.

LOCATION AND SELECTION OF THE APPROPRIATE INJECTION SITE

No one site can be recommended for all patients for ID, SC and IM injections. When selecting the appropriate site, the nurse must ensure the effectiveness of the medication. This is dependent on whether the drug reaches the intended site and is absorbed. Thus it is important to identify and select the appropriate anatomical site for ID, SC and IM injections and locate these accurately prior to giving an injection.

Intradermal

The most common sites for ID testing are the inner forearms and scapulae. If necessary, sites for SC injections can be used (Figure 10.1).

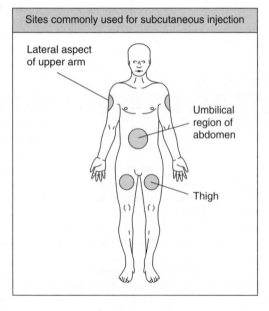

Fig 10.1 Sites commonly used for subcutaneous injections (Source: Hunter, 2008a; reproduced with kind permission of *Nursing Standard*)

Subcutaneous

Recommended sites are the lateral or posterior aspect of the lower part of the upper arm, the thighs (below the greater trochanter), the buttocks and the umbilical region of the abdomen. If necessary, the back and lower loins can also be used. The lower abdomen is the most common site of choice for administering heparin injections as this site has thicker SC tissue (Chan, 2001) (Figure 10.1).

Intramuscular

When choosing an appropriate site for administration, there are five sites that can be considered. Two recommended sites are the ventrogluteal and the vastus lateralis, which is a better choice for obese patients (Nisbet, 2006) (Figure 10.2).

The *mid deltoid site* is easily accessible. Only small volumes should be injected, up to a maximum of 1 ml. Due to the size of the muscle, the area should not be used repetitively (Rodger & King, 2000). The denser part of the deltoid must be located. To do this, imagine a triangle where the horizontal line is located 2.5–5 cm below the acromial process and the midpoint of the lateral aspect of the arm in line with the axilla forms the apex. The medication is then injected about 2.5 cm down from the acromial process. This avoids the radial and brachial nerves (Workman, 1999; Rodger & King 2000).

The *dorsogluteal site*, commonly referred to as the outer upper quadrant, is used for deep IM and Z track injections. A maximum of up to 4 ml can be injected into this muscle (Rodger & King, 2000). Usually this site is located by using imaginary lines to divide the buttocks into four quarters. However, to locate the gluteus maximus, visualise a line that extends from the iliac spine to the greater trochanter of the femur. Find the midpoint of the first line and draw a vertical line to identify the upper aspect of the upper outer quadrant. Accurate location avoids the superior gluteal artery and sciatic nerve (Workman, 1999; Small, 2004).

The *rectus femoris site* is the anterior quadriceps muscle and is used for deep IM and Z track injections. In adults, a volume of 1–5 ml can be injected, although for infants this would be 1–3 ml. The rectus femoris is a large and well-defined muscle and easily

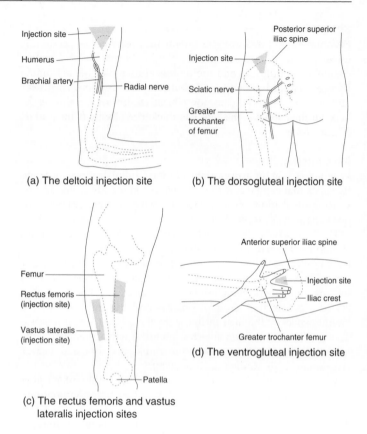

Fig 10.2 Sites commonly used for intramuscular injections. Reproduced from Rodger & King (2000), with permission of Blackwell Publishing Ltd

accessible. It is more likely to be used when individuals are self-administering injections or with children. It is located halfway between the superior iliac crest and the patella (Workman, 1999).

The *vastus lateralis site* is used for deep IM and Z track injections. Up to 5 ml can be injected into the muscle (Rodger & King, 2000). This muscle forms part of the quadriceps femoris group of muscles and is easily accessible. It is found on the outer side of the femur and can be located by measuring a hand's breadth from both the greater trochanter and the knee joint to clearly identify the middle third of the vastus lateralis muscle (Workman, 1999). This area is free from major blood vessels or structures that would cause an injury (Rodger & King, 2000).

The *ventrogluteal site* is the site of choice for deep IM and Z track injections, although the use of this site remains limited. Up to 2.5 ml can safely be injected into the muscle (Rodger & King, 2000). The site is located by placing the palm of the nurse's hand on the patient's opposite greater trochanter (e.g. the nurse's right palm on the patient's left hip). Then, by extending the index finger to the anterior superior iliac spine, a 'V'-shaped triangle is formed. The injection site is the centre of the 'V'-shaped triangle, the gluteus medius muscle (Rodger & King, 2000).

FACTORS TO CONSIDER WHEN SELECTING AN INJECTION SITE

When choosing an appropriate site for administration, the nurse will need to:

- inspect the skin surface. Areas of bruising, inflammation, oedema, lesions, scarring or infection should be avoided (Workman, 1999; Perry & Potter, 2006).
- consider if the patient is receiving regular SC injections. These should be rotated to avoid any irritation, scarring, hardening of the tissue and pain (Workman, 1999; Jamieson *et al.*, 2002; Nicol *et al.*, 2008; Shawyer & Endacott, 2009).
- consider the individual's physical condition and age and assess the amount of tissue available at a particular site. The amount of SC tissue available will vary. This could lead to the accidental administration of an SC injection into the muscle. In the case of insulin this will increase the rate of absorption, causing hypoglycaemia (King, 2003). With IM injections, choice will be influenced by the amount of muscle mass an individual has. Ideally, the muscle needs to be well vascularised and able to tolerate the required volume of solution. People who are active are more likely to have a greater muscle mass than

elderly or emaciated patients. If there is insufficient muscle mass, the tissues may need to be 'pinched' up prior to the injection (Workman, 1999; Rodger & King, 2000).

- assess the amount and type of medication to be injected, e.g. analgesic, antibiotic or depot injection;
- identify any factors that may restrict access, for example inability to move or may cause contamination of the site, e.g. wound dressing.

COMPLICATIONS ASSOCIATED WITH ID, SC AND IM INJECTIONS

The administration of any medication can pose a risk, therefore it is important to recognise and understand potential complications associated with injections. These include:

- Inappropriate selection of site and poor technique. This may lead to the inadvertent administration of an SC injection into the muscle, or an IM injection may go directly into a blood vessel. This will affect the rate and extent of absorption of the medication, increasing the risk of patient injury.
- Anaphylaxis; an allergic reaction caused by the medication, e.g. penicillin.
- Pain associated with local tissue damage caused by the speed at which medication is administered, volume of solution, needle size and poor technique (Torrance, 1989; Chan, 2001).
- Bruising associated with local tissue damage. This indicates local capillary bleeding in the dermal and SC layers of the skin. Probably most common with heparin injections (Chan, 2001).
- Nerve injury with the administration of IM injections. This ranges from foot drop to flaccid paralysis from sciatic nerve damage. It can also cause persistent leg and foot pain, and neuropathy (Rodger & King, 2000; Small, 2004).
- Sterile and septic abscesses associated with IM injections. These are caused when a large volume of solution is injected into a smaller muscle mass. This can lead to ischaemia and muscle necrosis (King, 2003).
- Muscle fibrosis and contracture. These occur when the same injection site is used for multiple injections. As with abscesses, if a large volume of solution is injected into a smaller muscle

mass this can cause ischaemia and muscle necrosis, leading to fibrosis and muscle contracture (Rodger & King, 2000).

• Necrosis and gangrene, which are more common in children. The combination of selecting an area of small muscle mass and using the incorrect needle size contributes to these complications, e.g. when the solution is injected into the lateral aspect of the mid-thigh (Watt, 2003).

PRINCIPLES OF PRACTICE FOR ADMINISTERING INJECTIONS

To ensure a safe standard of practice, nurses must be aware of and adhere to policies, procedures and guidelines issued by their organisation. This will state whether one or two nurses are required for the procedure. When administering medications, only registered nurses may administer these unsupervised. Student nurses must be directly supervised to facilitate safe knowledge and competent practice, and the registered nurse must countersign any documentation that is signed by the student nurse (NMC, 2008).

Patient preparation

Importantly, the nurse must explain the procedure so that the patient fully understands and is able to give his/her informed consent and cooperation. Information about the medication, action and side effects as well as the choice of site for the injection should be discussed. This allows the patient the opportunity to express any concerns and anxieties, and the patient's understanding can be evaluated. It is essential to check whether the patient has any known allergies to identify potential reactions to the medications (NMC, 2008, 2009).

The use of gloves and aprons

Before administering any injection, hands must be washed with an antimicrobial soap and dried thoroughly. This is also repeated immediately after the procedure. Gloves should be worn for all invasive procedures such as ID, SC and IM medication administration (Pratt *et al.*, 2007). Gloves help to prevent cross-infection and drug-induced allergies, but they do not protect the nurse from needlestick injury (Workman, 1999). Disposable aprons must be worn if close contact with the patient is anticipated and/ or if there is a risk of clothing being contaminated when preparing and administering the medication (Pratt *et al.*, 2007).

Skin cleaning

The practice of cleansing the injection site with an impregnated alcohol swab before parenteral injections reduces the number of pathogens that can be introduced into the skin when administering the injection (Workman, 1999), but this practice is inconsistent. For SC injections, it is not necessary to clean the skin because with repeated use of an alcohol swab the skin will harden. This will reduce the rate of absorption and will significantly, over time, reduce the choice of sites.

When preparing the skin for intramuscular injection the site is normally cleaned with a swab saturated with 70% isopropyl alcohol. The nurse should rotate the swab from the injection site to approximately 5 cm away from this point in a circular motion (Perry & Potter, 2006). This should be continued for 30 s and then the skin allowed to dry. If the injection is given before the skin is allowed to dry, it may allow entry of bacteria and cause local irritation. The patient may also experience pain as the alcohol is injected into the tissues (Springhouse Corporation, 1993).

Some organisational policies no longer consider skin cleansing necessary if the skin is physically clean [Wynaden *et al.*, 2005; Department of Health (DH) 2006] and the required standard of hand washing and asepsis is maintained (Workman, 1999). If the skin is visibly dirty, the injection site area will need to be cleaned to decontaminate the skin (Nicol *et al.*, 2008).

Needle size and angle of injection

Re-sheathing a needle *before* the medication is administrated to a patient is safe. This is achieved by using the aseptic non-touch technique as described by Nicol *et al.* (2008). This, prevents droplets of the medication from being sprayed onto the skin or inhaled when air is being expelled from the syringe (Nicol *et al.*, 2008).

ID route injections are given with a 25-gauge needle and inserted, bevel up, at an angle of 10–15°, just under the epidermis. As the drug is injected, a wheal appears on the skin surface (Perry & Potter, 2006).

Traditionally, SC injections have been given using an 'orange' or size 25-gauge needle for all adult patients. As the needle length is greater than 5–8 mm, injections are normally given at a 45° angle. However, with the introduction of shorter needles with pre-filled syringes and insulin 'pens', it is now recommended that injections are given at a 90° angle. This ensures that the medication is injected into the SC layer (King, 2003). Consideration to needle size and the angle of insertion is required when the patient is obese or cachectic. This is to ensure that injection is given into the SC adipose (fatty) tissue rather than into the muscle (IM) or just under the epidermis (ID).

When giving an IM injection, a 'green' or size 21-gauge needle is used for adult patients to ensure that the medication is injected into the muscle, at an angle of 90°, using a 'dart'-like motion until 0.5–1 cm of the needle is left showing (Nicol *et al.*, 2008). This also applies to patients who are cachexic or thin, except that the needle is not inserted as deeply. If a smaller gauge needle is used, the nurse needs more pressure to inject the solution, which will increase the patient's discomfort (King, 2003). Critically, the needle must be long enough to reach the muscle at the chosen site and, therefore, an assessment of the patient's muscle mass and SC fat is necessary to determine the right length of needle to use (Lenz, 1983; Perry & Potter, 2006). These range from 2.5 to 5.0 cm.

The Z track technique

Two methods are suggested for administering IM injections. One method is to stretch the skin over the chosen injection site to displace the underlying subcutaneous tissue, and the second method involves the 'Z track' technique. This technique causes less discomfort and prevents leakage from the needle site (Rodger & King, 2000).

This is achieved by pulling the skin 2–3 cm sideways or downwards from the injection site, which causes the skin and SC tissues to slide over the underlying muscle by 1–2 cm. Hold the needle at a 90° angle above the injection site, quickly pierce the skin in a dart-like motion until 1 cm of the needle is left. Aspirate for blood; if no blood is withdrawn, then slowly inject the medication and hold in place for 10 s. Withdraw the needle quickly. Finally, release the tension on the skin, which allows the tissues to return to their original position. This creates a disjointed pathway that seals the injection entry point. Medication is now unable to seep into the SC tissues or leak out through the injection site (Workman, 1999; Rodger & King, 2000; Jamieson *et al.*, 2002).

Equipment required
You will need the following equipment when administering injections:

- a prescription chart;
- the prescribed drug to be administered – depending on the route of administration, this may be a pre-filled syringe or the medication may be a single- or multidose preparation (Dougherty *et al.*, 2008);
- a clean tray or receiver;
- a syringe of appropriate size depending on the volume to be injected;
- the correct gauge needle;
- an alcohol-impregnated swab – IM injection only;
- a sterile, clinical wipe or tissue;
- a sharps container.

Preparation of the equipment

- Collect all the equipment. Check that all packaging is intact to retain sterility [National Patient Safety Agency (NPSA), 2007].
- Wash and dry hands thoroughly with an antimicrobial soap or use bactericidal hand rub to prevent any contamination of the equipment or medication. Put on gloves (Pratt *et al.*, 2007).
- Check the patient's prescription chart and determine the drug to be administered, required dose, route of administration, and date and time of administration. Check if the prescription is legible and signed by a doctor. These actions minimise any risk to the patient. If any errors are noticed withhold the medication and contact the medical team (NMC, 2008).

- If using a pre-filled syringe the following steps **will not** be necessary:
  - Prepare the medication:
    - Check the expiry date on all packaging. Discard the equipment if any packaging is damaged or has expired.
    - Open the packaging at the plunger end and remove the syringe. Ensure that the plunger moves freely inside the barrel; do not touch the nozzle end. Open the needle packaging at the hilt (coloured) end and attach the needle firmly onto the nozzle of the syringe. Loosen; but do not remove the sheath. Place the syringe and covered needle on the tray.
  - Examine the solution in the ampoule. Before breaking the neck of the ampoule with a clinical wipe or tissue, check that the contents are in the bottom of the ampoule. For plastic ampoules avoid touching the top of the ampoule with your fingers when breaking the top.
  - Pick up the syringe, allowing the sheath to fall off the needle into the tray. Insert the needle into the solution of the ampoule. Avoid scraping the needle on the bottom of the ampoule, as this will blunt the needle.
  - Pull back the top of the plunger using one finger on the flange to draw up the required dose into the syringe. If necessary, tilt or hold the ampoule upside down to make sure that the needle remains in the solution to prevent drawing in air.
  - Using the non-touch technique, carefully replace the sheath on the needle to maintain sterility.
  - Expel the air. Hold the syringe upright at eye level; let any air rise to the top of the syringe. Lightly tap the barrel to encourage any bubbles to rise to the top of the syringe. Push the plunger to expel the air until the solution is seen at the top of the needle.
  - **If using a pre-filled syringe, you should not expel the air from the syringe as the air bubble is designed to remain next to the plunger. When the medication is injected, the air fills the needle of the syringe so the whole dose is administered. Refer to the manufacturer's instructions for more information.**

Suggested procedure to administer the injection

- Take the prepared medication to the patient. Check the patient's name band according to local policy.
- Close the curtains around the bed or close the door to provide privacy and dignity. If necessary, adjust the bed height and assist the patient into a comfortable position. For IM injections, if the legs are slightly flexed the muscles relax. Expose the injection site but avoid leaving the patient exposed.
- For IM injections, clean the skin with an alcohol-impregnated swab.
- Prepare to inject the medication:
  - With ID injections, stretch the skin using the thumb and forefinger.
  - For SC injections, pinch the skin using the thumb and forefinger to lift the adipose tissue from the underlying muscle to prevent the solution from being injected into the muscle (King, 2003).
  - With IM injections, stretch the skin slightly over the chosen area to displace the underlying SC tissue to aid insertion. The Z track method can also be used (see page 215).
- Insert the needle smoothly at the correct angle.
  - For IM injections, slightly withdraw the plunger to confirm that the needle is in the correct position and has not entered a blood vessel. If blood is present, stop the procedure, withdraw the needle and recommence the procedure. If no blood is present continue with the procedure.
  - With ID and SC injections, it is not necessary to draw back on the plunger to ensure that the needle is not in the vein, as it is unlikely that a blood vessel will be pierced (McAskill & Goodhand, 2007; Nicol et al., 2008).
- Inject the solution by pushing carefully on the plunger. Wait 10 s before withdrawing the needle to allow the drug to diffuse into the tissues (Hunter, 2008b). For IM injections, the rate is 1 ml per 10 s (Workman, 1999; Dougherty et al., 2008).
- Use the tissue to wipe any fine capillary blood that might be leaking away. Do not massage the area as this may cause the drug to leak from the injection site and cause local irritation (Rodger & King, 2000).

- *Do not resheath the needle*. Discard the syringe and needle immediately into the sharps container to prevent any injury.
- Record the administration of the medication on the prescription chart to show that the drug has been given. Report any complications or adverse reactions (NPSA, 2007; NMC, 2008). Ensure that the patient is comfortable. Return to the patient after 15–20 min to evaluate the effectiveness of the medication. Return after 2–4 h to check the injection site (Rodger & King, 2000).
- Ensure that all equipment is disposed of safely.

CONCLUSION

The administration of injections is a valuable and necessary skill. This chapter has emphasised the principles of best practice along with a rationale to encourage safe practice. This requires the use of clinical judgement when choosing an injection site, and an understanding of the anatomical structures to prevent complications from occurring.

REFERENCES

Chan H (2001) Effects of injection duration on site-pain intensity and bruising associated with subcutaneous heparin. *J Adv Nurs* **35**(6): 882–892.

Corben V (2005) Administration of medicines. In: *Developing Practical Nursing Skills* (ed Baillie L), 2nd edn. Hodder Arnold, London.

Department of Health (DH) (2006) *Immunisation Against Infectious Disease – 'The Green Book'*. The Stationery Office, London.

Dougherty L, Farley A, Hopwood L, Sarpal N (2008) Drug administration: general principles. In: *The Royal Marsden Hospital Manual of Clinical Nursing Procedures* (eds Dougherty L, Lister S), 7th edn. Wiley-Blackwell, Oxford. pp. 202–253.

Greenway K (2004) Using the ventrogluteal site for intramuscular injection. *Nurs Stand* **18**(25): 39–42.

Hunter J (2008a) Subcutaneous injection technique. *Nurs Stand* **22**(21): 41–44.

Hunter J (2008b) Intramuscular injection techniques. *Nurs Stand* **22**(24): 35–40.

Jamieson EM, McCall JM, Whyte LA (eds) (2002) *Clinical Nursing Practices*, 4th edn. Churchill Livingstone, Edinburgh.

King L (2003) Subcutaneous insulin injection technique. *Nurs Stand* **17**(34): 45–52.

Lenz CL (1983) Make your needle selection right to the point. *Nursing* **13**(2): 50–51.

McAskill H, Goodhand K (2007) Administration of medicines. In: *Clinical Nursing Practices* (eds Jamieson EM, Whyte LA, McCall JM), 5th edn, Chapter 2. Churchill Livingstone Elsevier, Edinburgh. pp. 13–33.

National Patient Safety Agency (NPSA) (2007) *Promoting Safer Use of Injectable Medicines*. Alert No. 2007/20. 28th March. NPSA, London.

Nicol M, Bavin C, Bedford-Turner S, Cronin P, Rawlings-Anderson K (2008) *Essential Nursing Skills*, 3rd edn. Mosby, Edinburgh.

Nisbet AC (2006) Intramuscular gluteal injections in the increasing obese population: retrospective study. *Br Med J* **332**: 637–638.

Nursing & Midwifery Council (NMC) (2008) *Standards for Medicines Management*. NMC, London.

Nursing & Midwifery Council (NMC) (2009) *The Code: Standards of Conduct, Performance and Ethics for Nurses and Midwives*. NMC, London.

Perry AG, Potter PA (2006) *Clinical Nursing Skills and Techniques*, 6th edn. Elsevier Mosby, St Louis, Missouri.

Pratt RJ, Pellowe CM, Wilson JA, *et al.* (2007) Epic2: national evidence-based guidelines for preventing healthcare-associated infections in NHS hospitals in England. *J Hosp Infect* **65**(Suppl 1): S1–S64.

Rodger MA, King L (2000) Drawing up and administering intramuscular injections: a review of the literature. *J Adv Nurs* **31**(3): 574–582.

Shawyer V, Endacott R (2009) Drug administration. In: *Clinical Nursing Skills Core and Advanced* (eds Endacott R, Jevon P, Cooper S). Oxford University Press, Oxford. pp. 125–192.

Shepherd M (2002) Medicines 2. Administration of medicines. *Nurs Times* **98**(16): 45–48.

Small S (2004) Preventing sciatic nerve injury from intramuscular injections: literature review. *J Adv Nurs* **47**(3): 287–296.

Springhouse Corporation (1993) *Medication Administration and IV Therapy Manual*, 2nd edn. Springhouse, Pennsylvania.

Torrance C (1989) Intramuscular injection Part 1. *Surg Nurse* **2**(5): 6–10.

Watt S (2003) Safe administration of medicines to children: part 2. *Paediatr Nurs* **15**(5): 40–44.

Workman B (1999) Safe injection techniques. *Nurs Stand* **13**(39): 47–53.

Wynaden D, Landsborough I, Chapman R, McGowan S, Lapsley J, Finn M (2005) Establishing best practice guidelines for administering of intramuscular injections in the adult: a systematic review of the literature. *Contemp Nurse* **20**(2): 267–277.

Administration of Intravenous Fluids and Medicines

11

Dan Higgins

INTRODUCTION

Intravenous (IV) medicines administration is the process of administering a medicine directly into a patient's vein and consequently directly into their systemic circulation. Methods of administering IV medicine include rapid administration of relatively small volumes (bolus) into the vein using a syringe into an injection port, either on an administration set or directly into a vascular access device (VAD) such as a cannula (Shawyer & Endacott, 2009).

IV infusion administration is the process whereby IV medicines are given at controlled rates over a period of time, via gravity administration sets, volumetric infusion pumps or syringe drivers. For the purposes of this text, these two terms will be jointly called IV therapy.

IV therapy carries significant risk; the National Patient Safety Agency (NPSA) received 800 reports relating to injectable medicines between January 2005 and June 2006. This represents approximately 24% of the total number of medication incidents; within these reports there were 25 incidents of death and 28 incidents of serious harm (NPSA, 2007).

In order to comply with the Nursing & Midwifery Council (NMC) code (2008a), nurses must ensure that their practice with regard to the administration of IV medications is in line with local policies, as well as being undertaken in a safe, systematic and efficient manner. Doing so will ensure that the risks associated with such a route of administration are reduced. Nurses not only have to ensure that a medicine is administered as prescribed, but also that it is undertaken using professional judgment as outlined in the NMC document *Standards for Medicines Management* (NMC, 2008b).

Thus, therapy should be delivered according to the essential principles of safe drug administration as outlined in Chapter 6. Namely that medicines are:

- stored properly prior to use;
- administered to the right patient, who should receive the correct medicine at the correct dose and the correct formulation;
- delivered via appropriate route;
- administered at the correct time, at the correct rate, for the correct duration of therapy.

IV therapy is now an integral part of the majority of nurses' professional practice and can range from caring for an individual with a peripheral cannula in situ to nursing a patient requiring multiple parenteral drugs/infusions in the critical care environment [Royal College of Nursing (RCN), 2005].

IV drug administration is often associated with complications such as infections and phlebitis. Nursing staff will therefore have a responsibility to try and minimise the incidence of these effects, whilst at the same time ensuring that their patients receive their IV therapy in an appropriate and timely manner. Nursing staff are also responsible for evaluating and monitoring the effectiveness of a prescribed therapy, and documenting patient response, adverse events and any subsequent interventions (NMC, 2008b).

The aim of this chapter is to provide an overview of the administration of IV fluids and medicines.

LEARNING OUTCOMES

At the end of this chapter, the reader will be able to:

- ❏ List the indications for using the IV route.
- ❏ Discuss the complications associated with IV therapy.
- ❏ Demonstrate an understanding of the essential principles of IV drugs/fluid administration.
- ❏ Explain how nursing actions can minimise risks to patient safety.

❏ Outline the management of anaphylaxis.
❏ Discuss how the safe use of electronic infusion devices can be used to complement therapy.
❏ Demonstrate an understanding of some of the IV fluids used in a wide variety of clinical settings and the indications for use.

INDICATIONS FOR USING THE IV ROUTE

Medicines given intravenously avoid the process of absorption, resulting in immediate action (Galbraith *et al.*, 1999). This can have significant benefits, particularly in emergency care. The dose delivered is easy to control and the bioavailability, that is the amount of the unaltered medicine that reaches the circulation or site of intended action, is 100%. It is also easier to maintain drug blood levels to maintain therapeutic response (Lawson, 2009). Sustained therapeutic levels of a medication need to be maintained over a period of time through the use of a continuous infusion.

The immediate response associated with the IV route can be disadvantageous, as once administered there is an inability to recall the drug and reverse its action (Dougherty & Lister, 2008). The immediate availability of a medication may lead to increased risk of toxicity, since side effects are usually immediate and more severe.

The IV route may be of use where particular drugs are altered/inactivated by the gastrointestinal tract or metabolised in the liver before entering the systemic circulation (the hepatic first-pass effect). The vascular route affords a route of administration for patients who cannot tolerate fluids or drugs by the gastrointestinal route (Dougherty, 2002).

Some medicines are particularly irritant to tissues, therefore other routes of administration, such as intramuscular or subcutaneous, are unsuitable. When administered intravenously, these medicines are diluted by blood flow and are less likely to cause damage.

COMPLICATIONS ASSOCIATED WITH IV THERAPY

Complications associated with IV therapy include:

• anaphylaxis and acute reactions;
• embolus;

- infection risks;
- extravasation/infiltration;
- phlebitis;
- drug incompatibilities;
- risks associated with indwelling VADs.

Anaphylaxis and acute reactions

The term 'anaphylaxis' refers to a severe, life-threatening, gener-
alised or systemic hypersensitivity reaction [Resuscitation
Council (UK), 2008]. It can be brought about by a broad range of
triggers, but IV medicines, in particular antibiotics and anaesthetics, are common factors (Pumphrey, 2004). Anaphylaxis must be
considered a risk in all patients receiving IV therapy and systems
must be in place to ensure rapid emergency treatment, should it
occur.

The management of anaphylaxis is demonstrated in Appendix
11.1.

Rapid administration of IV medicines can also result in 'speed
shock', which differs from anaphylaxis in that it is a reaction to
a sudden increase in drug concentrations in the circulation.
Symptoms can include a flushed face, headache, chest tightness,
cardiac arrhythmias loss of consciousness and cardiac arrest.

Embolus

The risk of embolus formation may be related to the VAD and
thrombus formation around the device or may be a result of the
introduction of air or particulate matter into the circulation.
Nurses must be aware of the signs and symptoms of air embolus,
which may include:

- deteriorating levels of consciousness;
- acute cardiovascular collapse;
- acute respiratory failure.

If any of these symptoms are present, emergency treatment
should be initiated without delay.

Filter or 23-gauge needles are recommended for drawing up
from glass ampoules, to minimise the risk of injecting glass or

drug particles into patients (RCN, 2005). The medicine should always be carefully inspected for glass and particulate contamination prior to administration (Higgins, 2005). Air-in-line detectors should be used to monitor for air bubbles in administration sets when delivered via electronic infusion devices (RCN, 2005).

Infection risks

All patients receiving IV therapy are at an increased risk of developing either local or systemic infections, either through microbial contamination of the medicines or as a result of indwelling VADs. Infection should be suspected if signs and symptoms, such as redness or discharge at the IV site or an elevated temperature, develop.

All IV therapy should be managed according to guidelines outlined in *The Royal College of Nursing Standards for Infusion Therapy* (RCN, 2005), and simple evidence-based tools such as Saving Lives High Impact Interventions care bundles (www.clean-safe-care.nhs.uk). The use of aseptic non-touch techniques (ANTT) for IV therapy preparation is becoming popular across many NHS organisations. The ANTT is a proven, evidence-based method used to standardise aseptic technique. It is a simple, efficient and logical approach to IV therapy and is the same for both peripheral and central line access (University College London Hospitals, 2007).

Extravasation/infiltration

Extravasation is defined as the inadvertent administration of vesicant medication or solution into the surrounding tissue instead of into the intended vascular pathway (RCN, 2005). This can lead to severe local tissue damage, resulting in delayed healing, infections and possibly tissue necrosis. The term 'vesicant' describes medicines that can cause necrosis to tissues.

Extravasation can occur through misplacement or dislodgment of the VAD; this is frequently seen in patients with poor venous networks. The treatment of extravasation should be prompt and must include discontinuation of the therapy and immediate intervention undertaken as outlined by local policy.

Tissue infiltration occurs when a non-vesicant solution leaks into the surrounding tissue and usually occurs as a consequence of improper placement or dislodgment of the cannula.

Phlebitis

Phlebitis, or inflammation of the vein, is a common complication of IV therapy. It may occur as a result of the indwelling VAD or it may be related to the concentrations of the infused/injected medicines. Nurses should ensure that drugs are reconstituted according to the sources listed above and reconstitution is carried out in a manner that avoids infusion of particles. All vascular access sites should be routinely assessed for signs and symptoms of phlebitis using the Vein Infusion Phlebitis Scale (VIP) (Jackson, 1998; RCN, 2005).

Drug incompatibilities

There is a risk of harm to the patient through medicine incompatibility where multiple drugs are used or during the reconstitution process. An incompatibility can manifest as a visible reaction such as colour change, haze, turbidity, precipitate or gas formation, or it could be chemical where there is non-visible degradation of the drug (Dougherty, 2002). If at all possible, medicines should be prepared in closed, not open, systems, which ensures greater accuracy and sterility in the preparation of IV medications (Dougherty, 2002; NPSA, 2007).

Advice regarding both the incompatibility and medicine stability, once reconstituted, can be found on the product data sheet in the medicine packaging or via the *British National Formulary* [British Medical Association (BMA) & Royal Pharmaceutical Society of Great Britain (RPSGB), 2009]. If this information is not readily available, the advice of a pharmacist should be sought.

Risks associated with indwelling VADs

Specific management of VADs is beyond the scope of this text, but practice should be informed by the guidelines above and nursing care should be directed to reducing the transmission of infection and the incidence of VAD complications.

Fluid overload

This can occur as a result of the volumes of fluid that are required to reconstitute certain medicines. Even if these volumes are given over long time periods, the patient should be assessed for signs of cardiovascular compromise. As a minimum standard, all hospitalised patients receiving IV therapy should have fluid balance measurement recorded and vital sign observations on a regular basis.

INFUSION SYSTEMS AND THE USE OF ELECTRONIC INFUSION DEVICES IN IV THERAPY

An infusion system is the process by which an infusion device and any associated disposables are used to deliver fluids or drugs in solution to the patient via the IV, subcutaneous, epidural, parenteral or enteral route (Medical Devices Agency, 2003). An infusion device (Figure 11.1) enables the delivery of a medicine or fluid to a patient at a constant rate over a set period of time to achieve a desired therapeutic response (Dougherty & Lister, 2008).The simplest infusion systems are gravity administration sets, which use gravity and a roller clamp mechanism to gauge the rate of an infusion. Whilst having advantages, volumetric accuracy cannot be guaranteed (Dougherty & Lister, 2008).

Electronic devices are now commonplace; the use of powered infusion devices has grown enormously in the last 20 years and they have moved from being tools to support clinical practice to being an integral requirement in treatment delivery (Quinn, 2000). These devices vary from simple volumetric peristaltic pumps to syringe drivers capable of delivering small fractions of volume. Universally, the use of any of these devices appears to carry a significant risk of error, many of these resulting in patient harm or death.

The Medical Devices Agency, now the Medicines and Healthcare products Regulatory Agency (MRHA), has outlined specific recommendations with regard to the use of infusion devices:

- A clearly defined structure for the management of infusion systems must exist within a trust.

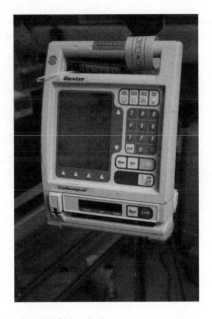

Fig 11.1 Example of an IV infusion device

- A suitable medical device coordinator(s) should take responsibility for the management of infusion systems. This coordinator will have specific responsibilities, including policy development, maintenance, staff training and responding to safety warnings.
- Adverse incidents should be reported.

Nursing responsibilities when caring for patients with infusion devices are based around competency with the specific device and comprehensive patient assessment. Staff should ensure that they have received training on the particular device and their competency has been assessed. This is becoming somewhat easier, as many organisations have rationalised the range and types of infusion devices. The overall safety mechanism is one of patient and device monitoring.

The use of gravity infusion sets appears to be in decline for larger volumes of fluid, although their use is common for small volume (<100 ml) antibiotic/medicine therapy or infusions considered to carry low risk. Because of variation in flow, patients receiving therapy in this way should be monitored closely. Nurses must ensure that they are competent in the formulae to calculate infusion rates for both electronic devices and gravity administration; these are outlined in Chapter 6.

IV FLUID THERAPY

IV fluid therapy is the administration of volumes of greater then 100 ml into a vein (Lawson, 2009). This is performed on a bolus, intermittent or continual basis. IV fluid therapy may be undertaken to replete or maintain the hydration status of a patient. It may also be used as a carrier mechanism for medicines or to replace depleted circulating substances such as electrolytes. The decision to hydrate a patient has traditionally been the domain of medical staff, but, with the advent of nurse prescribing, these clinical decisions are now often made, and treatment initiated, by nurses.

Patients who cannot meet their nutrition needs using normal or enteral mechanisms may receive IV nutrition. Administration of such fluid is beyond the scope of this text. Blood is not classified as a medicinal product, although some blood components are (NMC, 2008). In this text, transfusion of blood and blood products is not discussed in any depth.

The basis for commencing IV fluids will be made following comprehensive assessment of the patient and their fluid status. Fluid replacement therapy is also indicated in patients who are at risk of becoming dehydrated. The type of fluid that patients will require will be dependent on their history and clinical presentation and responses to any therapy. The differing classes of fluid replacement therapies are outlined in Box 11.1.

The safe principles outlined for IV therapy above are relevant for fluid therapy; the additional associated risks are predominantly related to under- or over-hydration and metabolic/electrolyte derangement. All patients receiving IV fluids must be monitored closely and, as a minimum, this should include fluid

---

Box 11.1 Parenteral preparations for fluid and electrolyte imbalance

Parenteral preparations for fluid and electrolyte imbalance consist of a combination of electrolytes in water or plasma and plasma substitutes.

Electrolytes in water (crystalloid solutions)

These are given to meet normal and electrolyte requirements or to replenish substantial deficits or continuing losses when the patient is nauseated, vomiting or unable to take adequate amounts orally (BMA & RPSGB, 2009).

The type of solution will be prescribed based on the patient's individual needs and may vary over a course of treatment. This decision will be based on comprehensive patient assessment and biochemical/haematological investigations. Solutions may be hypotonic, isotonic or hypertonic. Hypertonic solutions are ideally administered via large (preferable central) veins.

Plasma and plasma substitutes (colloid solutions)

Plasma and plasma substitutes contain large molecules that do not readily leave the intravascular space, where they exert an osmotic pressure to maintain circulatory volume (BMA & RPSGB, 2009). The large molecules may be prepared from whole blood, dextrans, starches or gelatine.

These solutions are used frequently in fluid resuscitation as it is thought that a lower total volume of fluid is required, as fluid will be 'pulled' from the extracellular compartments.

Plasma and plasma substitutes are often used in very ill patient whose condition is unstable, therefore close monitoring is required and fluid and electrolyte should be adjusted to the patient's condition at all times (BMA & RPSGB, 2009).

Adapted from BMA & RPSGB (2009).

balance measurement, vital signs observation and biochemical/ haematological assessments.

SUGGESTED GUIDELINES FOR IV MEDICINE AND FLUID ADMINISTRATION

These guidelines are suggestions only; nurses should ensure that they practice within organisational policy. All nurses who administer IV therapy must have received approved training and undertaken supervised practise. The onus is also on the individual to ensure that knowledge and skills are maintained both from a theoretical and a practical perspective.

It is important to bear in mind that an injectable medicine must not be prepared too far in advance of its administration nor should it be prepared by anyone other than the individual who is to administer it.

Checklist for the preparation and administration of an IV medication (for example powdered antibiotics)

- Check the medication to be administered against the prescription, which should contain the approved medicinal name, dose to be administered, route, and date and time(s) of administration. For the prescription to be legally valid, it must be signed by the prescriber. Should there be any ambiguity regarding the prescription, clarification should be sought before proceeding any further.
- Ascertain the properties of the medicine to be administered, seeking advice as necessary. Nurses must employ their professional judgement in all cases of medicine administration, knowing the indications for, the pharmacokinetics of and the usual dosage of the medicine along with any side effects and contraindications (Trounce, 2000).
- Perform any required mathematical calculation of dosage and rate of infusion. Some drug administrations can require complex calculations to ensure that the correct volume or quantity of medication is administered; in such cases, it is good practice for a second practitioner to check the calculation independently in order to minimise the risk of error (NMC, 2008).
- Check the above with another registered practitioner as required by organisational policy. Wherever possible two

registrants should check medication to be administered intravenously, one of whom should also be the nurse who then administers the medication (NMC, 2008).

- Undertake an assessment of the patient and perform any baseline observations as required.
- Explain the possible risks and benefits to the patient. This forms part of informed consent, which must be obtained. The NMC recommends that treatment plans involving medication are undertaken wherever possible with the full informed consent of the person receiving the drugs (NMC, 2008).
- Wash hands. Don clean apron. Apply any other personal protective equipment as required.
- Prepare all equipment according to local policy, ensuring hand hygiene and employing the ANTT where appropriate.
- Prepare/reconstitute the drug as per the manufacturer's instructions/local policy. Care must be taken to avoid excess positive and negative pressures within the medicine vial; this can be achieved by reconstituting the drug using a venting needle or by injecting small volumes of air into the vial to displace the reconstituted drug.
- Air should be expelled from the syringe; this is best achieved by disposing of the aspiration needle, positioning the syringe with the luer connector uppermost. The syringe plunger can then be pulled fully back to allow air to move to the top of the syringe. Tap the syringe to dislodge any air bubbles. The air can then be expelled by depressing the syringe plunger. This process should not be performed with the needle on the syringe, as aerosols may be created.
- Correctly identify the patient (as outlined in Chapter 6).
- Administer the drug as prescribed.
- Date and initial the relevant parts of the prescription sheet.
- If the medication is withheld for any reason, this should be documented on the prescription chart and in the nursing notes. It may be prudent in most cases to inform a clinician (NMC, 2008).

Procedure for fluid-filled glass ampoules

The procedure for administration of medicines from glass ampoules is the same as that outlined above. The top of the ampoule may need to be tapped to allow any trapped drug to drain into the bottom of the ampoule. The ampoule top may then be covered with sterile gauze/pad and snapped, using a dot marker as a guide if appropriate (Higgins, 2005). The solution should be inspected for cloudiness or particulate matter, both before and after snapping the ampoule neck (Dougherty & Lister, 2008).

Procedure for powder-filled glass ampoules

The procedure for administration of powdered medicines from glass ampoules will follow the same principles as above. The hydrolysis of the powder cake should be done slowly to avoid medicine wastage/aerosol formation.

Procedure for administering IV fluids via gravity administration sets or device-specific administrations sets

As for IV medications, but the key differences are as follows:

- Ensure that the bag of fluid is not contaminated in any way and that the solution resembles the normal characteristics as outlined in the product information. Also make sure that fluid separation or precipitation has not occurred.
- Remove any protective packaging and, using an aseptic technique, snap the seal where the administration set trocar is to enter the bag (this may require inverting the bag if semi-rigid containers are used). If possible hang the fluid on a drip stand (Higgins, 2004) (Figure 11.2).
- Close any flow controllers on the administration set, expose the trocar and advance into the appropriate port.
- Gently squeeze the drip chamber, allowing it to partly fill with fluid.
- Partially release the flow controller to allow fluid to fill and move through the tubing. This may require removing the protective cap at the luer lock connector to allow air to be expelled.
- Expel any air particles by allowing the fluid to run through the set into a receptacle. Replace the protective cap and connect to the patient's intravascular device according to local policy.

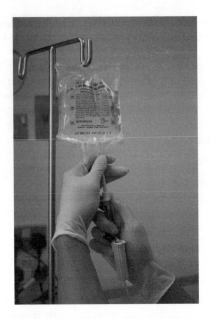

Fig 11.2 IV fluid therapy: ideally use a drip stand

Important points to note:

- If using glass containers, an air inlet will be required to equalise pressure in the bottle, thus facilitating the flow of fluid (Jamieson *et al.*, 2002).
- If using an electronic infusion device, the administration set should be primed according to the manufacturer's recommendations.
- The administration of any medicines using central venous access devices and that of parenteral nutrition is subject to specific guidelines not discussed in this text.

CONCLUSION

The use of IV medications is part of everyday nursing practice in both primary and secondary care settings. There are many indications for using the IV route in medicine administration and use of the route appears to be becoming increasingly common. However, IV therapy continues to be associated with a relatively high risk of complications; many of these are not predictable, specifically adverse reactions such as anaphylaxis. However, the majority of complications can be prevented through ensuring that certain standards in nursing practice are maintained. Nurses must ensure that practice is informed, evidence based and underpinned by sound knowledge of the medicines being administered, their pharmacokinetics, and the use of the IV route and its alternatives.

Technological advances mean that health care is now complemented/complicated by an increasing amount of electronic and computer-controlled devices. Nurses must ensure that they are competent in the use of such technology in order to reduce risk to the patient receiving the therapy.

Whilst all risk cannot be negated, nurses should also be prepared to respond to adverse events should they occur and not only deliver care in response to this, appropriately and efficiently, but also use these experiences to improve patient safety.

IV therapy goes hand in hand with VADs and the care of such. In order to minimise risks to patients, nurses must use the same evidence-based approach to care when using such devices to ensure effective care and therapy.

APPENDIX 11.1 ANAPHYLAXIS ALGORITHM

Anaphylaxis algorithm

Anaphylactic reaction?

Airway, Breathing, Circulation, Disability, Exposure

Diagnosis - look for:
- Acute onset of illness
- Life-threatening Airway and/or Breathing and/or Circulation problems[1]
- And usually skin changes

- **Call for help**
- Lie patient flat
- Raise patient's legs

Adrenaline[2]

When skills and equipment available:
- Establish airway
- High flow oxygen
- IV fluid challenge[3]
- Chlorphenamine[4]
- Hydrocortisone[5]

Monitor:
- Pulse oximetry
- ECG
- Blood pressure

[1] **Life-threatening problems:**

Airway:	swelling, hoarseness, stridor
Breathing:	rapid breathing, wheeze, fatigue, cyanosis, SpO_2 < 92%, confusion
Circulation:	pale, clammy, low blood pressure, faintness, drowsy/coma

[2] **Adrenaline** *(give IM unless experienced with IV adrenaline)*
IM doses of 1:1000 adrenaline (repeat after 5 min if no better)
- Adult — 500 micrograms IM (0.5 mL)
- Child more than 12 years: 500 micrograms IM (0.5 mL)
- Child 6 – 12 years: 300 micrograms IM (0.3 mL)
- Child less than 6 years: 150 micrograms IM (0.15 mL)

Adrenaline IV to be given **only by experienced specialists**
Titrate: Adults 50 micrograms; Children 1 microgram/kg

[3] **IV fluid challenge:**
Adult - 500 – 1000 mL
Child - crystalloid 20 mL/kg

Stop IV colloid if this might be the cause of anaphylaxis

	[4] Chlorphenamine (IM or slow IV)	[5] Hydrocortisone (IM or slow IV)
Adult or child more than 12 years	10 mg	200 mg
Child 6 – 12 years	5 mg	100 mg
Child 6 months to 6 years	2.5 mg	50 mg
Child less than 6 months	250 micrograms/kg	25 mg

Reproduced by permission of the Resuscitation Council.

REFERENCES

British Medical Association & Royal Pharmaceutical Society of Great Britain (2009) *British National Formulary*. BMJ Publishing Group Ltd, London, and RPS Publishing, London.

Dougherty L (2002) Delivery of intravenous therapy. *Nurs Stand* **16**(16): 45–52.

Dougherty L, Lister S (2008) *The Royal Marsden Hospital Manual of Clinical Nursing Procedures*, 7th edn. Wiley-Blackwell, Oxford.

Galbraith A, Bullock S, Mainias E, Hunt B, Richards A (1999) *Fundamentals of Pharmacology: A Text for Nurses and Health Professionals*. Pearson Prentice-Hall, Harlow.

Higgins D (2004) Priming an IV infusion set. *Nurs Times* **101**(47): 32–33.

Higgins D (2005) IV drug preparation and reconstitution. *Nurs Times* **101**(47): 22–23.

Jackson A (1998) A battle in vein infusion phlebitis. *Nurs Times* **94**(4): 68–71.

Jamieson EM, McCall J, Whyte LA (2002) *Clinical Nursing Practices*, 4th edn. Churchill Livingstone, Edinburgh.

Lawson C (2009) Administering intravenous fluids. In: *Clinical Nursing Skills, Core and Advanced* (eds Endacott R, Jevon P, Cooper S). Oxford University Press, Oxford.

Medical Devices Agency (2003) *Infusion Systems Device Bulletin*. DB 9503. Medical Devices Agency, London.

National Patient Safety Agency (NPSA) (2007) *Patient Safety Alert 20: Promoting Safer Use of Injectable Medicines*. NPSA, London.

Nursing & Midwifery Council (NMC) (2008a) *The Code: Standards of Conduct, Performance and Ethics for Nurses and Midwives*. NMC, London.

Nursing & Midwifery Council (NMC) (2008b) *Standards for Medicines Management*. NMC, London.

Pumphrey RS (2004) Fatal anaphylaxis in the UK, 1992–2001. *Novartis Found Symp* **257**: 116–128.

Quinn C (2000) Infusion devices, functions and management. *Nurs Stand* **14**(26): 35–41.

Resuscitation Council (UK) (2008) Emergency treatment of anaphylactic reactions – Guidelines for healthcare providers. Available at www.resus.org.uk/pages/reaction.pdf [accessed in October 2009].

Royal College of Nursing (RCN) (2005) *Standards for Infusion Therapy*. RCN, London.

Shawyer V, Endacott R (2009) Administering an intravenous injection. In: *Clinical Nursing Skills, Core and Advanced* (eds Endacott R, Jevon P, Cooper S). Oxford University Press, Oxford.

Trounce J (2000) *Clinical Pharmacology for Nurses*. Churchill Livingstone, Edinburgh.

UCLH (2007) *UCLH Injectable Medicines Administration Guide*, 2nd edn. Blackwell Publishing, Oxford.

Miscellaneous Routes of Medication Administration

12

Matthew Aldridge

INTRODUCTION

In this chapter, miscellaneous routes of drug administration that nurses may be expected to undertake will be discussed. It should be remembered that at all times when engaging with drug administration, nurses should act in accordance with the Nursing & Midwifery Council's standards for medicines management guidelines [Nursing & Midwifery Council (NMC), 2008]. Practitioners must also remember that additional local standards for measuring competency in medication administration may apply, and in this case to ensure that they have been deemed competent in administration of medication by a particular route by their employer if necessary.

It is vital that nurses have an understanding of the pharmacological actions, side effects, cautions and contraindications of any medicine they are administering and, if in any doubt, to seek clarification by consulting any or all of the following: the current version of the *British National Formulary* (BNF), the prescriber of that medicine, pharmacist, doctor or a senior colleague.

In all cases of medication administration, good assessment is vital to establish a history with regard to indications for a drug and any allergies to medications. The registered nurse must ensure that he or she follows the common steps as identified by the Department of Health [Department of Health (DH), 2004] to ensure the safer administration of medications, often referred to as the five Rs of drug administration:

- *Right patient*: by ensuring that you check patient identification wristbands and challenge name, date of birth, etc. against the prescription chart.

- *Right drug*: check packaging, details of prescription – clarify with the BNF, prescriber or other sources as described above if necessary.
- *Right dose*: check packaging and prescription as above. Ensure correct calculation by using appropriate formulae and check with colleague if necessary.
- *Right route*: check prescription, packaging and indication for the patient's condition.
- *Right time*: check prescription and the BNF for indicated frequencies, i.e. once every 6h or twice daily.

The aim of this chapter is to provide an overview of miscellaneous routes for drug administration.

LEARNING OUTCOMES
At the end of this chapter, the reader will be able to:

❏ Describe the administration of topical drugs (local and systemic).
❏ Describe the administration of medication via the ear.
❏ Describe the administration of medication via the eye.
❏ Describe the administration of medication via the nasal route.
❏ Describe the administration of inhaled medication.
❏ Describe the administration of medication per rectum.
❏ Describe the administration of medication per vagina.
❏ Describe the administration of medication via the sublingual and buccal routes.
❏ Describe the administration of medication via the intraosseous route.
❏ Describe the administration of medication via the intrathecal route.

ADMINISTRATION OF TOPICAL DRUGS (LOCAL AND SYSTEMIC)
There are a large number of commercially available products available both on prescription and over the counter that are designed to be administered topically. The application of topical medication is intended to allow a medication to be absorbed into the epidermis (outer layer of the skin) and external mucous membranes (Bailie, 2005).

The range of topical medications can be broadly categorised into creams, lotions, ointments and powders (Greenstein & Gould, 2004). Topical medications that are intended to have a systemic effect, for instance glyceryl trinitrate (GTN) patches, are also considered to be topical by nature of their route of administration.

Topical medications with a local effect are often used to treat skin conditions, such as eczema, or localised infections. Common examples included hydrocortisone cream and fucidic acid.

Topical medications with a systemic effect are often referred to as 'transdermal medications', and are commonly used in the form of an adhesive patch impregnated with a particular medication. This route of administration can be beneficial in a number of ways: the drug bypasses the gastrointestinal system so is less likely to cause gastrointestinal upset; the patient does not have to remember to take multiple doses, as per the oral route, and effect is often long acting, so eliminates the need for frequent application or replacement (Greenstein & Gould, 2004). This route can be particularly useful in providing a sustained, slow release of a drug into a patient's system with minimal interference or discomfort to the patient, for instance pain relief in a palliative care situation.

Professional considerations

Even though topical medications are often considered to be easier to administer with fewer side effects than other routes, it is important that nurses recognise that the application of a topical medication is still subject to the same administration guidelines as drugs administered via any other route. Subsequently, topical administration should only be carried out by a registered practitioner competent in medication administration or healthcare students who are under the direct supervision of such a registered practitioner.

Technique

- Wash hands and don non-sterile disposable gloves if applying creams or ointments.
- Explain and discuss procedure with the patient.

- Check the five Rs of medication administration with the patient, prescription chart and packaging.
- Check for broken skin (some topical medications may be contraindicated if the patient has broken skin, whereas some topical drugs may actually be indicated to treat the condition causing the broken skin).
- If the medication is to be rubbed into the skin then a sterile topical swab should be used, as opposed to the nurse's finger or hand, in order to minimise cross-infection and exposure to the drug by the person administering the drug (Dougherty & Lister, 2008).
- Advise the patient if the medication is likely to cause staining of either the skin or fabrics, so that the patient can act accordingly with re-clothing.
- Document administration and wash hands.
- When applying transdermal patches to the same patient on an ongoing basis, it is important to rotate the site of application to prevent skin irritation or breakdown. Always remove the previous patch if replacing with a new patch of the same medication, in order to prevent multiple dosing (Perry & Potter, 2006).

ADMINISTRATION OF MEDICATION VIA THE EAR

Medication administered via the ear is most commonly in the form of installation of ear drops that can be used to soften wax before syringing, reduce inflammation or combat infection (Jamieson *et al.*, 2007). Drugs administered via this route are intended to have a localised effect and act within the anatomy of the ear and auditory canal.

Professional considerations

As mentioned with topical medications, ear drops should only be administered by registered practitioners competent in medication administration or healthcare students who are under the direct supervision of such a practitioner.

Technique

- Wash hands.
- Explain and discuss procedure with the patient.

- Check the five Rs of medication administration with the patient, prescription chart and packaging.
- Ask the patient to lie on their side with the affected ear uppermost, or if not possible to lie down, to tilt their head to do so.
- Warm drops to body temperature if possible to minimise discomfort during administration (Dougherty & Lister, 2008).
- Pull the pinna (outermost part) of the ear gently in an upward and backward direction in adults, and a downward and backward direction in children in order to straighten the external ear canal and ensure that drops are directed towards the eardrum (Jamieson *et al.*, 2007).
- Instil the required number of drops in the ear (Figure 12.1).
- Ask the patient to try and remain in the same position for 1–2 min to allow absorption (Dougherty & Lister, 2008).
- Record administration of medication and wash hands.

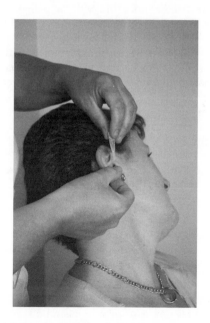

Fig 12.1 Administration of a medication via the ear

ADMINISTRATION OF MEDICATION VIA THE EYE

Drops or ointments administered via the eye are commonly used to treat localised infection or inflammation and can also be used to supplement or substitute secretions from tear ducts.

Professional responsibilities

As mentioned with topical medications, ear drops should only be administered by registered practitioners competent in medication administration or healthcare students who are under the direct supervision of such a practitioner. Always apply drops before ointment if both are prescribed, as ointment will leave a film on the eye, which may hamper the absorption of medication in drop form.

Technique – eye drops

- Wash hands.
- Explain and discuss procedure with the patient.
- Check the five Rs of medication administration with the patient, prescription chart and packaging.
- It is preferable for ease of administration that the patient should lie supine, looking upwards, but if this is not possible then the patient should be seated with their head tilted back and supported.
- The patient should be encouraged to look upwards and the drops should be instilled onto the lower lid of the eye rather than directly onto the globe, as this will aid retention of the medication (Marsden & Shaw, 2003) (Figure 12.2).
- The patient should also be encouraged to close the eye for 60 s after instillation to aid retention and absorption (Bailie, 2005).

Technique – ointment

- Wash hands.
- Explain and discuss procedure with the patient.
- Check the five Rs of medication administration with the patient, prescription chart and packaging.
- It is preferable for ease of administration that the patient should lie supine, looking upwards, but if this is not possible

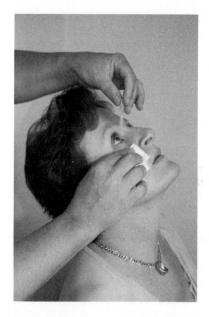

Fig 12.2 Administration of eye drops

then the patient should be seated with their head tilted back and supported.

- Evert the lower lid by applying and pulling down on the lower lid with a wet swab.
- Whilst holding the ointment tube 2.5 cm above the eye, gently squeeze the tube to release the medication in a line across the inner edge of the lower lid (Dougherty & Lister, 2008).
- Advise the patient that their vision may be blurred for a short time after administration, and to refrain from driving or operation of machinery until their vision returns to normal.

ADMINISTRATION OF MEDICATION VIA THE NASAL ROUTE

Medications administered via the nasal route are commonly used to treat conditions such as allergic rhinitis, and can offer relief of symptoms of nasal congestion or rhinorrhoea. Medications may take the form of nasal sprays or drops.

Professional responsibilities

As mentioned with topical medications, nasal drops or sprays should only be administered by registered practitioners competent in medication administration or healthcare students who are under the direct supervision of such a practitioner.

Technique

- Wash hands.
- Explain and discuss procedure with the patient.
- Check the five Rs of medication administration with the patient, prescription chart and packaging.
- It is preferable for ease of administration that the patient should be lying supine, looking upwards for the installation of drops, or seated upright with the head slightly forward for the installation of nasal sprays (Burns, 2007).
- Encourage the patient to clear their nostrils by blowing or manually cleaning with a tissue or damp cotton bud to ensure that the drug has access to the nasal mucosa (Dougherty & Lister, 2008).
- For drops, instil the required number of drops into the nostril(s) as required.
- For sprays, ensure that the pump action of the spray is primed if required. If the patient is unable to self-administer the medication, insert the nozzle into nostril whilst occluding the opposite nostril with a finger. The patient should be encouraged to gently inhale through the nostril whilst the pump spray is activated.
- The procedure should be repeated for the other nostril if appropriate.
- The patient should be discouraged from sniffing too vigorously post administration, as this can cause 'run-off' from the medication down the nasopharynx, which can cause an unpleasant taste in the throat and affect absorption of the medication (Burns, 2007).

ADMINISTRATION OF INHALED MEDICATION

Drugs administered via the inhaled route are primarily concerned with the treatment of respiratory disorders, such as asthma and chronic obstructive pulmonary disease (COPD). The benefit of this route of administration is the deposition of the inhaled drug into the bronchial tree, where its intended pharmacological action takes place, although studies suggest that when drugs are inhaled via pressurised metered dose inhalers (PMDIs), only approximately 10% of an inhaled dose actually makes it further into the respiratory system than the larynx (Currie & Douglas, 2006). This is why correct administration technique is particularly important, as incorrect technique will diminish the amount of drug reaching the bronchial tree further still.

Drugs administered via the inhaled route include β_2-agonists such as salbutamol and salmeterol acting as a bronchodilator. Corticosteroids such as beclomethasone, which suppress inflammation, are also often prescribed to asthmatics who have more frequent exacerbations of asthmatic conditions.

Inhalers

Some patients, particularly the elderly and children, can often find the technique required for administration of an inhaler difficult, as a certain level of dexterity is required in simultaneous actuation and inhalation to administer the dose. However, this can be made easier by the use of a spacer device (Figure 12.3) or chamber that holds the medication inside until inhalation can take place. A spacer eliminates the need for the simultaneous actuation and inhalation of the medication.

Professional responsibilities

Good administration technique is vital when using inhaled medication, and because often this type of medication is self-administered by patients it is the nurse's role to offer appropriate patient education in the correct technique when using inhalers.

There are many different versions of PMDIs available, with differing methods of actuation, therefore it is important to refer to the manufacture's instructions before offering advice on correct use of a device.

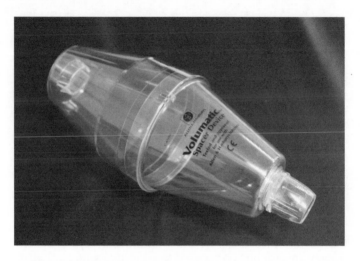

Fig 12.3 Spacer device

Technique

- Wash hands.
- Explain and discuss procedure with the patient.
- Check the five Rs of medication administration with the patient, prescription chart and packaging.
- Ask the patient to remove the mouthpiece cover from the inhaler.
- Ask the patient to shake the PMDI and then breathe out.
- Advise the patient to place the mouthpiece into their mouth and close their lips and teeth around it.
- Encourage the patient to actuate the spray whilst inhaling simultaneously (Figure 12.4).
- Ask the patient to remove the inhaler from their mouth and to hold their breath for 10s if possible (Jevon & Humphrey, 2007). The patient should continue to breathe normally for 1min before repeating a further dose.
- If a spacer device is to be used, then the patient should connect the PMDI to the spacer device, actuate the spray and then inhale from the spacing device (Figure 12.5). In infants and

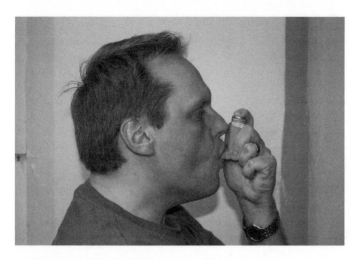

Fig 12.4 Administration of a medication using an inhaler

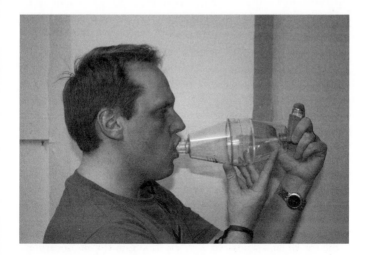

Fig 12.5 Using a spacer device

children under the age of 2 years, a mask should be attached to the mouthpiece of the spacer device in order to facilitate its effective use (Jevon & Humphrey, 2007).

Nebulisers

A nebuliser (Figure 12.6) can be described as a device that converts a liquid into a fine spray (Muers, 1997), and the aim of this device is to deliver particles that are small enough to reach the bronchioles, notably to administer a larger therapeutic dose of a drug within a period of 5–10 min (British Thoracic Society, 2004). Nebulisers require a source of gas to force the medication into mist form (jet-driven) (Figure 12.6a) or can be driven ultrasonically using sound waves to agitate the medication into mist form (Figure 12.6b). In the majority of cases, nebulisers are commonly jet-driven via compressed air from either a cylinder or a compressor box. For patients who are having an acute asthma attack, nebulisers should be driven via oxygen to prevent desaturation (Jamieson *et al.*, 2007).

Nebulisers are often used in the treatment of acute asthma for the administration of short-acting β_2-agonists such as salbutamol but can also be used to administer medications in long-term conditions such as COPD. Certain medications, such as corticosteroids, may cause irritation around the lips or mouth when given regularly via the nebulised route. In this case, it may be more beneficial to use a mouthpiece rather than a mask to deliver the medication.

Technique

- Wash hands.
- Assemble required equipment.
- Explain and discuss procedure with the patient.
- Check the five Rs of medication administration with the patient, prescription chart and packaging.
- Ensure that the patient is sitting as upright as possible to effective inhalation.
- In patients with asthma requiring administration of a bronchodilator, obtain a peak expiratory flow rate (PEFR) recording prior to commencement (Rees & Kanabar, 2006).

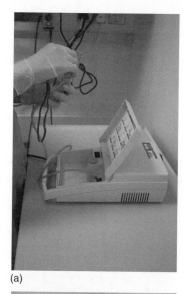

(a)

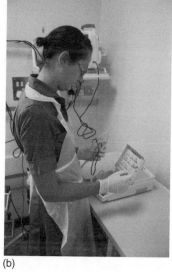

(b)

Fig 12.6 Nebulisers

- Unscrew the chamber of the nebuliser device and transfer medication into the reservoir. Reassemble the chamber when done.
- Attach air/oxygen supply as prescribed and appropriate to the nebuliser device.
- Attach mask or mouthpiece as appropriate and fit the mask to the patient or ask them to hold the mouthpiece.
- If using a piped air or oxygen supply, ensure that the flow rate is set to 6–8 l/min to ensure effective nebulisation of the medication.
- Once misting has finished, discontinue nebuliser (Jevon & Humphrey, 2007) and, if appropriate and prescribed, recommence any ongoing oxygen therapy at the appropriate dose.
- Wash and dry the nebuliser chamber if to be reused (remember that these devices are for single patient use only).
- Repeat PEFR recording if appropriate.
- Document and wash hands.

ADMINISTRATION OF MEDICINES PER RECTUM

Indications
The rectal mucosa, whilst having a small surface area, has a relatively large vascular supply and is able to facilitate rapid absorption of medications (Richardson, 2008). Another advantage of giving drugs via this route is that the liver is bypassed, therefore absorption of drugs that may be affected or destroyed by the liver can be given successfully via the rectal route. Drugs commonly administered via this route can be divided into those that have a topical effect and those that are intended to have a systemic effect.

Topical
Rectal suppositories, such as glycerin, and enemas, for example sodium phosphate, are administered for the relief of constipation and are designed to act within the rectum, loosening the passage of faeces. Preparations for the treatment of haemorrhoids such as local anaesthetic cream combined with hydrocortisone are also administered rectally in order to have a topical effect within the rectum and around the anus.

Systemic

Diazepam is given for the control of seizures. Administering a benzodiazepine via this route is particularly useful, as obtaining intravenous access in a fitting patient can be difficult and dangerous, and training to administer diazepam via this route can also be offered to patients' carers, who may have to deal with fits outside of the clinical area.

Anti-inflammatory drugs such as diclofenac can be administered rectally for the relief of musculoskeletal pain, thereby reducing the risk of gastric irritation that exists when using this medication orally.

Prochlorperazine administered as an anti-emetic can be given rectally and is particularly useful if patients are unable to tolerate oral medications due to nausea and vomiting.

Paracetamol as an anti-pyretic can be administered rectally and is fast acting when given via this route.

Professional responsibilities

Administration of medication by the rectal route can be embarrassing and uncomfortable for the patient. It is the nurse's responsibility to ensure that patient's dignity and comfort is maintained wherever possible during administration of a rectal medication. Patients must be informed if possible of the alternatives, as not all patients may be willing to receive medication via this route.

Side effects of drugs administered rectally

With all medication administered rectally there is the possibility of local anal or rectal irritation. Inflammation of the rectum can occur and, more rarely, perforation of the colonic mucosa.

Technique
Suppositories

The nurse should always check the five Rs of medication administration before administering any medication.

- Explain the procedure to the patient and obtain consent.
- Wash hands and obtain the appropriate equipment (Pegram *et al.*, 2008):
  - prescription chart;
  - suppositories as prescribed;

- non-sterile disposable gloves and apron;
- disposable waterproof sheet;
- tissues or gauze;
- receiver;
- water-based lubricant;
- clinical waste bag.

- Ensure that the patient's privacy and dignity are considered by drawing curtains around the bed space and place a water-proof sheet between the patient and the bed linen to prevent soiling, whilst minimising exposure of the patient by covering the patient with a sheet and only removing garments as necessary. In order to facilitate easy insertion of the suppository, it is accepted that the ideal position for the patient is the left lateral position, i.e. the patient lying on their left-hand side with their knees drawn up to their chest.

- The nurse should part the patient's buttocks and visualise the anus, first inspecting for any abnormalities that may make suppository insertion difficult, such as haemorrhoids. The presence of blood noted per rectally should be a contraindication to suppository insertion, and the nurse should abort the procedure and seek medical review for the patient.

- If no contraindications exist, then the nurse should lubricate the end of the suppository to be inserted with a small amount of water-based lubricant. Pegram *et al.* (2008) suggest that the suppository should be inserted blunt-end first to facilitate easier insertion and aid retention.

- Insert the suppository using the first or second finger to guide it under direct visualisation. This is particularly important when performing the procedure on a female patient to avoid accidental vaginal administration of the medication.

- Following insertion of the suppository, wipe around the patient's anus to remove any excess lubricant and ensure that the patient is in a comfortable position. If the suppository is for the relief of constipation, then encourage the patient to retain it for at least 15–30 min. If the suppository is to be retained in order to administer a medication, then encourage the patient to try and refrain from passing faeces for at least 30 min post insertion.

- If the suppository is for the relief of constipation, ensure that the patient has adequate access to toilet facilities or the call bell if they are unable to self-mobilise.
- Dispose of waste and record the administration of the suppository on the patient's prescription chart and notes.

ADMINISTRATION OF MEDICATION PER VAGINA

The vaginal route of medication is commonly used for the treatment of localised vaginal infections of a bacterial or fungal nature. Vaginal medication usually comes in the form of pessaries (similar in shape and nature to a suppository) or in a pre-loaded applicator.

The same protocols for checking the five Rs of medication administration and promoting patient privacy and dignity as per rectal administration should be followed. The patient can be encouraged to adopt either the left lateral position or the supine position with the knees drawn up and the legs parted to aid insertion (Dougherty & Lister, 2008). Consideration should be given, where possible, to allowing the woman to administer the medication herself or for the nurse to assist her in doing so.

Technique

- Wash hands and don gloves and protective apron.
- Check the five Rs of medication administration with the patient, prescription chart and packaging.
- Locate the vagina (it is important to visualise the vagina to prevent inadvertent insertion of the medication into the anus).
- Gently insert the pessary or pre-loaded applicator as far into the vagina as comfortable. If using a pre-loaded applicator, it will be necessary to push the plunger fully to administer the medication. Withdraw the applicator, if used, when dose is administered.
- Wipe away any excess medication and offer the patient a pad to protect their underwear from any leakage of medication.
- Encourage the patient to remain on their side or back for as long as possible. It is often best to administer vaginal medication last thing at night so that the patient can remain in bed to

minimise leakage of medication post administration (Nichol *et al.*, 2004).

ADMINISTRATION OF MEDICATION VIA THE SUBLINGUAL AND BUCCAL ROUTES

Sublingual medications are placed in the oral cavity under the tongue, whereas buccal medications are designed to be held in the cavity between the cheek and the molar teeth (Clayton *et al.*, 2007). The main advantages of these routes of administration are rapid absorption and avoidance of metabolism by the liver. Drugs commonly administered via this route include GTN for the treatment of angina and anti-emetics such as prochlorperazine.

Professional responsibilities

Medicines by this route are often self-administered by patients, therefore correct administration technique is vital. The nurse has a role to ensure that patients are educated in the correct administration technique. It is important that patients are instructed not to swallow drugs intended for sublingual or buccal administration, as digestion into the gastrointestinal tract will affect absorption and subsequently the action of the medication.

Technique

- Discuss administration with the patient and answer any questions the patient may have.
- Check the five Rs of medication administration with the patient, prescription chart and packaging.
- If possible, allow the patient to place the medication themselves under the tongue (sublingual) or between the upper molar teeth and the cheek (buccal). If the patient is unable to do this then use a gloved hand to place the medication.
- Advise the patient not to swallow the medication and not to eat, drink or swallow excessively until the medication has dissolved.
- If concurrent medication administration is to take place via the oral and sublingual/buccal routes, for example aspirin and GTN, administer the oral medication before the sublingual/

buccal to avoid inadvertent swallowing of medication not designed for the oral route.
- Remove gloves/wash hands and document administration appropriately.

ADMINISTRATION OF MEDICATION VIA THE INTRAOSSEOUS ROUTE

Intraosseous (IO) administration consists of the infusion of a drug or fluid into the medullary cavity of a bone through a specialised cannula, known as an IO device (O'Shea, 2005). This method of administration has become the route of choice when no other source of central access can be obtained to deliver drugs and fluid replacement in an emergency scenario and is more common in paediatric patients [Resuscitation Council (UK), 2006], although it can also be considered with adults if no other forms of rapid access for drug delivery are available (Proehl, 2004). Sites of choice often include the tibial plateau and medial malleolus, and in adults it is possible to use the sternum, but this can present problems if the patient then requires chest compressions as part of cardiopulmonary resuscitation.

Professional responsibilities

The insertion of an IO device (Figure 12.7) should only be carried out by an experienced, registered practitioner who has been deemed competent in using this technique. The insertion of an IO device should be avoided if the patient has any of the following: fracture (or suspected fracture) of a bone at the intended insertion site, burns over the intended insertion site, or conditions such as osteoporosis or osteogenesis imperfecta.

Technique

- Insertion of an IO device should preferably be preceded by administration of a local anaesthetic to minimise patient discomfort. This step may be omitted in cardiac arrest and critically ill patients if time does not allow.
- Once the needle has been inserted by a qualified, competent practitioner, it should be secured as appropriate, and, if possible, the limb should be immobilised using a splint to prevent unnecessary movement.

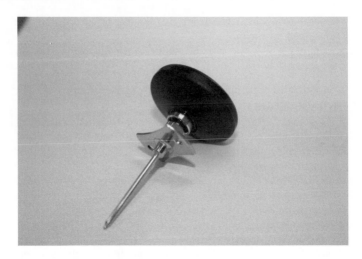

Fig 12.7 Intraosseous device

- The infusion should be established following the same aseptic non-touch technique as for an intravenous infusion.
- The infusion site should be closely monitored for fluid leakage or swelling, and any infusion should be discontinued and medical review sought immediately (Proehl, 2004).

ADMINISTRATION OF MEDICATION VIA THE INTRATHECAL ROUTE

Administration of drugs via the intrathecal route involves injection of fluid directly into the central nervous system. This is achieved by passing a needle through the theca, which surrounds the spinal column, thus allowing drugs to be injected into the subarachnoid space, through which cerebrospinal fluid circulates around the brain and spinal column (Greenstein & Gould, 2004). Drugs administered intrathecally include local anaesthetics, chemotherapy agents and antivirals.

Caution

There have been 55 known cases worldwide to date involving maladministration of chemotherapy drugs via the intrathecal route, resulting in death or paralysis of a patient (DH, 2008). Many of these cases result from the inadvertent intrathecal administration of a drug designed to be given only by the intravenous route. An example of this is the intravenous vinca alkaloid chemotherapy agent vincristine, which when administered intrathecally can cause paralysis and death.

Professional responsibilities

Intrathecal administration of medication must only be carried out by trained practitioners who have been assessed as safe and competent to do so by their employer. Significant harm can be caused by maladministration of drugs via the intrathecal route, and all necessary checks and safety precautions must be undertaken before commencing any intrathecal therapy. Local policies and guidelines should always be consulted and followed prior to commencement of any medication via the intrathecal route. It is the nurse's responsibility to ensure that local policies, procedural guidelines and safety checks are properly carried out when assisting with intrathecal procedures.

Technique

- Ensure that the procedure has been explained to the patient and that they are aware of any risks and offer appropriate consent.
- The use of correct aseptic non-touch technique is vital when carrying out insertion of intrathecal needles and administration of medication via the intrathecal route to minimise risk of infection.
- The nurse should prepare the appropriate equipment for lumbar puncture or insertion of intrathecal device if necessary.
- Chemotherapy drugs should be prepared by a registered pharmacist and only collected when required. The majority of hospitals forbid the storage of chemotherapy agents in the clinical area for safety reasons.
- Local policy for the safe administration of intrathecal medication should always be followed.

CONCLUSION

This chapter has provided an overview of miscellaneous routes for drug administration. The administration of topical drugs (local and systemic) and medications administered via the ear, eye and nose have been discussed. The administration of inhaled medication, medication per rectum and medication per vagina has been outlined. The administration of medication via the sublingual, buccal, intraosseous and intrathecal routes has been discussed.

REFERENCES

Bailie L (2005) *Developing Practical Nursing Skills*. Hodder Arnold, London.

British Thoracic Society (2004) *Guideline on the Management of COPD in Adults in Primary and Secondary Care*. BMJ Publishing Group, London.

Burns D (2007) Use of nasal sprays in allergic rhinitis. *Nurs Times* **103**(37): 24–25.

Clayton B, Stock Y, Harroun R (2007) *Basic Pharmacology for Nurses*. Mosby, St Louis, MO.

Currie G, Douglas J (2006) ABC of COPD: oxygen and inhalers. *BMJ* **333**: 34–36.

Department of Health (DH) (2004) *Building a Safer NHS for Patients, Improving Medication Safety: a Report by the Chief Pharmaceutical Officer*. HMSO, London.

Department of Health (DH) (2008) Updated national guidance on the safe administration of intrathecal chemotherapy. Health service circular 2008/001.

Dougherty L, Lister S (2008) *Royal Marsden Hospital Manual of Clinical Procedures*. Blackwell, London.

Greenstein B, Gould D (2004) *Trounce's Clinical Pharmacology for Nurses*, 17th edn. Churchill Livingstone, Edinburgh.

Jamieson E, Mcall J, Whyte L (2007) *Clinical Nursing Practices*, 5th edn. Elsevier, London.

Jevon P, Humphrey N (2007) Respiratory procedures: use of a nebuliser. *Nurs Times* **103**(34): 24–25.

Marsden J, Shaw M (2003) Correct administration of topical eye treatment. *Nurs Stand* **17**(30): 42–44.

Muers M (1997) Overview of nebuliser treatment. *Thorax* **52**(Suppl 2): S25–S30.

Nichol M, Bavin C, Bedford-Turner S, Cronin P, Rawlings-Anderson K (2004) *Essential Nursing Skills*. Mosby, London.

Nursing & Midwifery Council (NMC) (2008) *Standards for Medicines Management*. NMC, London.

O'Shea R (2005) *Principles and Practice of Trauma Nursing*. Elsevier, Oxford.

Pegram A, Bloomfield J, Jones A (2008) Safe use of rectal suppositories and enemas with adult patients. *Nurs Stand* **22**(38): 38–40.

Perry A, Potter P (2006) *Clinical Nursing Skills and Techniques*. Elsevier, Mosby, St Louis, MO.

Proehl J (2004) *Emergency Nursing Procedures*, 3rd edn. Saunders, St. Louis, MO.

Rees J, Kanabar D (2006) *ABC of Asthma*. Blackwell, Oxford.

Resuscitation Council (UK) (2006) *Provider Manual for Use in the UK: European Paediatric Life support Course*, 2nd edn. Resuscitation Council (UK), London.

Richardson R (2008) *Clinical Skills for Student Nurses: Theory, Practice and Reflection*. Reflect Press, Exeter.

13 | Medicines Management in Children

Elizabeth Payne

INTRODUCTION

Medicines management is 'the clinical, cost effective and safe use of medicines to ensure patients get the maximum benefit from the medicines they need, while at the same time minimising potential harm' [Nursing & Midwifery Council (NMC), 2007; National Prescribing Centre, 2000]. Children form one of the largest groups of patients consulting GPs and hospital healthcare professionals. The use of medicines is the most common therapeutic intervention carried out in the NHS.

Children's bodies respond to medicines differently from those of adults, and young children differently from older children. Thus, prescribers need to take into account age, weight and developmental stage when prescribing any medication for children. Lack of evidence on the use of medicines in children leads to uncertainty in dosing and, even at the most appropriate dose, may lead to differences in effectiveness and adverse effects as compared to those seen in adults.

When most new medicines are licensed or receive their marketing authorisation, they are only licensed for use in adults. The *informed* use of unlicensed medicines or of medicines for unlicensed applications (off-label use) is thus often unavoidable for children if they are to have access to the most effective medicines. Lack of formulations of licensed medicines for children frequently necessitates the use of products made for adults, and hence the need for the calculation of doses and accurate measurement of small liquid dose volumes; this increases the risk of error in prescribing and administration.

Evidence suggests that medication safety needs to be improved, particularly in babies and young children. Errors in prescribing and administration of medicines to children are at least as common as in adults. However, the consequences of these errors can be more serious.

The National Service Framework for Children, Young People and Maternity Services (2004) established clear standards for promoting the health and well-being of children and young people and for providing high-quality services that meet their needs. These standards form the basis of a 10-year plan to improve health care in children. One of the standards relates to medicines and states that:

> *Children, young people, their parents or carers, and health care professionals in all settings make decisions about medicines based on sound information about risk and benefit. They have access to safe and effective medicines that are prescribed on the basis of the best available evidence.*

The aim of this chapter is to understand medicines management in children.

LEARNING OUTCOMES

At the end of this chapter, the reader will be able to:

❏ Discuss the factors affecting drug disposition in children.
❏ Outline the principles of prescribing in children.
❏ Discuss medication safety in children.

FACTORS AFFECTING DRUG DISPOSITION IN CHILDREN

An understanding of the wide variability and constant changes in pharmacokinetic (what the body does to the drug) handling and the pharmacodynamic (what the drug does to the body) response to drugs, which occurs from the time of birth to adulthood, is essential in ensuring safe and effective drug treatment in children; these changes account for many of the differences in drug doses at various stages of childhood. In particular, special care is needed in the neonatal period, when the risk of toxicity is greater because of inefficient renal filtration, relative enzyme deficiencies, differing target organ sensitivity and inadequate detoxifying systems, which cause delayed excretion.

Practical problems in drug absorption, distribution, metabolism and excretion result from the altered pharmacokinetic handling of medicines seen at different stages of childhood development (NPC, 2000; Conroy 2003; SNAPP).

Absorption

The oral route of administration is the route of choice. However, drug absorption is dependent on gastrointestinal function, which changes rapidly after birth. During the first 6 months of life, peristalsis and gastric emptying are relatively slow and dependent on gestational and postnatal age, feeding patterns and the nature of the feed. Reduced production of bile results in reduced solubilisation of fat-soluble drugs. Variable rates of colonisation by gut microflora, high levels of β-glucuronidase activity in the gut, spitting out of medicines and vomiting all add to variable and unreliable absorption of oral medicines. Nevertheless, some drugs can be given successfully to babies tolerating milk feeds, such as caffeine solution for apnoea.

At birth, gastric pH is between 6 and 8, and remains relatively high until gradually falling to adult levels by the age of 2–3 years. A relatively high gastric pH occurs in the premature neonate, whose immature gastric mucosa leads to reduced acid secretion, which can lead to increased absorption of acid-labile drugs, such as penicillin, because of reduced drug breakdown. Increased or decreased absorption of weakly acidic or basic drugs can occur because of changes in ionisation state, e.g. slowed or reduced absorption of acidic drugs such as phenytoin, phenobarbitone and rifampicin.

The intramuscular (IM) route is not only painful but also unpredictable in premature infants due to low muscle mass, reduced variable blood flow throughout muscle tissue, inefficient muscle contractions and vasomotor instability (exaggerated vasoconstrictor reflex). Hence, the IM route should be avoided if possible.

Neonates and children have a large body surface area relative to body weight and well-hydrated skin. As a result, transdermal absorption is greatly increased. Where there is difficult venous access and unreliable oral absorption, the transdermal route offers an alternative route of administration but may also lead to greater risk of toxicity. Indeed, neurotoxicity and death have occurred from hexachlorophene through increased drug absorption. Also, potent topical steroids can lead to systemic adverse effects such as adrenal suppression and even Cushing's syndrome, particularly if the skin is broken or burnt. Further research is needed to produce drugs that may be administered transdermally without increasing the risk of toxicity.

The rectal route of administration may be an option if oral and intravenous (IV) administration is not possible, e.g. diazepam rectal tubes for status epilepticus. However, there is considerable variation in individuals' blood supply to the rectum, causing variation in the rate and extent of absorption of rectally administered drugs. Furthermore, suppositories containing appropriate doses for infants and children may not be available. As a result, nursing staff may need to administer a fraction of a suppository and thus a different dose to that intended, since distribution of the active ingredient in the suppository base is uneven.

Distribution

Total body water is much higher in neonates and children than in adults, for example 92% in the premature neonate compared with 75% in the newborn baby and 60% in small children; extracellular water follows a similar pattern, with 50% available in newborns, reducing gradually to 25% in a 1-year-old child. As a result, medicines such as gentamicin, distributed extensively into extracellular water, result in significantly increased volumes of distribution in neonates and young infants, and larger loading doses per kilogram may be required to achieve therapeutic concentrations.

Plasma protein concentration, binding affinity and capacity are reduced in the neonate. Furthermore, high bilirubin concentrations may cause drug displacement from plasma proteins; this is of particular concern in neonatal jaundice. Highly protein-bound drugs such as furosemide and phenytoin are significantly less protein bound in neonates than in adults, which results in increased volumes of distribution and levels of free drug. Hence, larger loading doses of highly protein-bound drugs may be needed in neonates to produce the desired serum concentration.

Metabolism

The main site of drug metabolism is the liver. At birth, clearance rates of drugs metabolised by the liver may be reduced as a result of immature liver enzyme processes, therefore extended dose intervals or reduced doses are necessary. For example, once-daily dosing of phenobarbital is adequate in a newborn baby, since its impaired metabolism in the first few days of birth results in a half-life of 70–200 h. (The duration of action of a drug is known as its half-life. This is the period of time required for the concentration or amount of drug in the body to be reduced by one half.) Twice-daily dosing becomes necessary by 2–3 weeks of age because the half-life reduces to 20–50 h and because there is liver enzyme induction as a result of the phenobarbital use.

Alternatively, some drugs may be metabolised by a different metabolic pathway, which is more advanced at birth than the pathway usually used in older children and adults. For example, paracetamol is metabolised by sulphation because this process is more advanced than the glucuronidation process, which is usual in older children and adults and takes several months to mature. Similarly, theophylline is metabolised by a different pathway in the newborn, resulting in caffeine production; caffeine is also active and so a lower dose is needed in the newborn.

In older children, hepatic function is greater than in adults. Most anti-epileptic and theophylline drugs require a larger dose per kilogram than adults to achieve therapeutic plasma concentrations. This is thought to be due to the fact that, relative to body size, the liver is larger than in adults.

Excretion

Renal excretion is the most important parameter that affects dosing of children at any age. Renal excretion is much reduced in newborn babies because it is dependent on glomerular filtration and tubular secretion, which is much reduced in babies. This persists until about 1 year of age. Hence, the clearance of renally excreted drugs, such as penicillins or aminoglycosides such as gentamicin, is much reduced in infants and particularly in preterm babies; as a result of this, extended dose intervals or reduced doses are necessary for renally excreted drugs.

Conversely, patients with cystic fibrosis are able to clear aminoglycosides at a much higher rate than normal children of the same age. The reasons for this have never been fully explained, but theories include enhanced tubular secretion, increased extra-renal clearance and increased volume of distribution. These patients nearly always require much higher doses of aminogly-cosides to achieve therapeutic plasma concentrations.

PRINCIPLES OF PRESCRIBING IN CHILDREN

Unlicensed and off-label medicines

Medicines must have a product licence (now called marketing authorisation) before being marketed in the UK to demonstrate that they are safe, effective and of a suitable quality. The product licence includes the indication, dose, route of administration and age group of patients for which the drug may be used.

Some medicines that are given to children are either:

- not licensed for use in children or are used outside the terms of their product licence (*off-label* use); or
- not licensed for any indication or age group (*unlicensed*).

The safety, efficacy and quality of these medicines for children can therefore not be guaranteed. Unlicensed and off-label pre-scribing does not imply inappropriate prescribing but reflects the lack of available evidence to support the use of these medicines in children – both in the formulations that children can take and in the appropriate dose ranges required (NPC, 2000; Morkane *et al.*, 2007; SNAPP).

There is a need to improve the provision of paediatric informa-tion in the manufacturers' product data sheet or summary of product characteristics (SPC). Many manufacturers write dis-claimers in the SPC stating that their products should not be used in children such as, 'contra-indicated in children' or 'insufficient information to recommend use in children', or make recommen-dations limiting them to specific age groups, indications or routes of administration. This can make it difficult for health profession-als to make informed decisions on the risk:benefit ratio of using a medicine for a particular indication, and even to identify whether or not it is licensed for use in children.

Use of a disclaimer also avoids the need to perform the studies required to support a paediatric licence application. Clinical trials are more expensive and time-consuming to conduct in children because of ethical, practical and technical problems. The commercial benefit to manufacturers of licensing a drug in the relatively small paediatric market is not seen as being sufficient to justify these extra costs. The economic reality is that trials are not conducted and drugs are not licensed.

On the other hand, a licence does not necessarily mean that a product is 'good' to prescribe. There is no evidence that most licensed cough medicines are any more effective than placebo and, potentially, they all have side effects. It is believed that only about half of the facts about a drug are known at the time of licensing. It follows that the use of licensed drugs is not without its problems, and post-marketing surveillance has a crucial role to play in achieving safe and effective medication use.

Licensing arrangements constrain pharmaceutical companies but not prescribers. The Medicines Act 1968 and European legislation make provision for doctors to prescribe, pharmacists to dispense and nurses to administer unlicensed medicines or medicines in an off-label capacity. However, individual prescribers are always responsible for ensuring that there is adequate information to support the quality, efficacy, safety and intended use of a drug before prescribing it.

UK and US paediatric professional bodies' statements stress that unlicensed and off-label drug use is a vital part of paediatric therapeutics. The best information available should be used to inform practice, and such practice should be in accordance with a respectable, responsible body of professional opinion. It is now considered that a prescriber could be subject to claims of malpractice if he/she denied a patient the best potential treatment just because it was unlicensed or off-label.

Some health authorities suggest that GPs should not prescribe unlicensed or off-label drugs. However, it may be difficult to continue supply from distant hospitals. Other health authorities suggest that patients should be told if the drug is unlicensed or off-label and even recommend that written consent is obtained before starting treatment. Paediatric professionals advise that it is not necessary to obtain additional consent from parents/carers/patients to prescribe or administer such drugs, over and above that obtained for other prescribed drugs.

Extent and nature of unlicensed and off-label medicine use in children

The extent of unlicensed and off-label drug use in children has been extensively documented and is known to be widespread, as demonstrated by UK studies [Scottish Neonatal and Paediatric Pharmacists Group (SNAPP)] and reflected by studies in other countries, which show that at least one unlicensed or off-label drug is received by:

- 90% of babies in neonatal intensive care;
- 70% of patients in paediatric intensive care;
- 67% of children in hospitals across Europe;
- 11% children treated at home by their GP.

The situations where unlicensed medicines have to be used when no appropriate licensed formulation of a drug is commercially available include:

- *Extemporaneous dispensing*: This often involves crushing tablets or opening capsules and suspending the contents to produce a formulation that a child can take in appropriate strengths for the paediatric or neonatal dose, e.g. clobazam suspension. This manipulation of the licensed dose form changes the product into an unlicensed product.
- *Purchase of unlicensed formulations*: Purchase of unlicensed products from a 'specials' pharmaceutical manufacturer means that these preparations may be prepared under good manufacturing conditions and may have undergone quality assurance processes. They will not, however, have been through clinical trials to determine the indications and dose regimens for their use, e.g. caffeine oral solution and injection.
- *Purchasing of drugs licensed in other countries*: Drugs that are licensed in other countries but not in the UK may be imported, e.g. vitamin A drops from Italy. There is great variation between countries as to product availability; the process of

importation is complicated, and as a result the product may be expensive.

- *'Named patient' supplies*: Pharmaceutical companies may occasionally supply unlicensed drugs on a 'named-patient' basis, e.g. captopril liquid.
- *Use of chemicals*: This may be necessary to treat rare conditions for which there is no licensed preparation or pharmaceutical-grade material available, e.g. isosorbide is used to treat hydrocephalus.

The situations where a drug is used off-label, i.e. use outside the conditions of the product licence or marketing authorisation, include:

- *Dose*: The dose may need to be lower or higher than recommended depending on the age and weight of the child, as drug handling capacity is constantly changing through the developmental stages of life. For example, the licensed dose of gentamicin in preterm babies results in subtherapeutic post-dose levels, and potentially toxic levels before subsequent doses are given due to reduced elimination. An off-label dose is therefore recommended to ensure effective therapy without toxicity.
- *Age of patient*: Drugs are often not licensed in children under a certain age, or for any children, even if they are commonly used, e.g. oral morphine solution is not licensed for use in children under the age of 1 year.
- *Indication*: Drugs may be used to treat childhood illnesses not covered by the licence. Diclofenac is used orally to treat pain in post-operative children, but it is licensed only for juvenile idiopathic arthritis.
- *Route of administration*: Alternative routes of administration may be necessary in children. For example, cyclizine injection is licensed only for IV or IM administration in adults. IM injections are avoided whenever possible in children, and therefore cyclizine is given by subcutaneous injection in some centres.
- *Contraindications*: These may need to be disregarded. Aspirin is used in Kawasaki disease, for example, despite being contra-indicated in children under the age of 16 years.

Practical problems due to lack of licensed medicines for children

Stability of an extemporaneously prepared medicine
Little information may be available on the bioavailability of the drug or the physical, chemical and microbial stability of the preparation when preparing a suitable medicine extemporaneously. This may result in a product that is unpleasant to take or has a short shelf life.

Supply of an extemporaneously prepared medicine
Maintaining supplies of an extemporaneously prepared medicine on discharge of a child from hospital may be problematic and may result in a delay or break in treatment. Problems can be avoided by prompt communication between hospital and community pharmacists in sharing dose and formulation information and ingredient sources or in arranging preparation by a 'specials' manufacturer.

Excipients
The availability of a product in a suitable dosage form is not an indication of its suitability for children. Some commercially available products contain excipients inappropriate for consumption by children such as alcohol, propylene glycol, dyes, colourings and E numbers. For example, if a 5 ml (15 mg) dose of a commercially available formulation of phenobarbital elixir containing 38% alcohol was given to a 3 kg baby, this would be equal to an adult swallowing a couple of glasses of wine.

An EC directive, issued in 1997, stated that 'benzyl alcohol is contraindicated in infants/young children'. Benzyl alcohol has been associated with a fatal toxic syndrome in preterm neonates, and therefore parenteral preparations containing the preservative should not be used in neonates. Both amiodarone and lorazepam injections contain benzyl alcohol, and both SPCs state that these products are contraindicated in infants or young children up to 3 years old. This poses a dilemma, given the lack of more appropriate alternatives for these patients.

The sugar content of medicines must also be considered, particularly with long-term treatment; it is unlikely to be a major issue in short-term medication. Sugar-free preparations should be used where available to help prevent dental caries. A variety of alternative sweetening agents such as aspartame, sorbitol, glycerol, xylitol, maltitol, mannitol, etc. are used in place of sucrose, glucose or fructose but can cause problems in some patients. Aspartame should be used with caution on phenylketonuria because of the phenylalanine content; sorbitol may produce diarrhoea if large doses are given.

Lack of patient information leaflets

Patient information leaflets (PILs) have been shown to improve concordance, and pharmacists are legally obliged to provide them with dispensed medicines. However, they are not usually available for patients taking unlicensed medicines. They are also not applicable for off-label medicines, as the information will relate to the licensed use. They are therefore likely to be confusing and may cause unnecessary worry. Counselling by a doctor or pharmacist who is aware of this issue should allay fears. However, many doctors and pharmacists are unaware when the prescriptions they write or dispense are off-label.

The Neonatal and Paediatric Pharmacists Group (NPPG) and the Royal College of Paediatrics and Child Health (RCPCH) have produced a general PIL about unlicensed or off-label medicines in children, which is available on www.nppg.org.uk. Furthermore, the NPPG and RCPCH, in conjunction with the national children's charity WellChild, have produced a series of PILs (further PILs are to follow) directed at the specific information needs of parents/carers and children and the conditions/illnesses for which they are prescribed, which are available on www.medicinesforchildren.org.uk/medicines/index.php.

Adverse drug reactions

Unanticipated adverse drug reactions (ADRs) are probably the greatest concern created by the use of unlicensed and off-label drugs. Age-dependent changes in pharmacokinetics and pharmacodynamics may not be known when a drug is used in an unlicensed or off-label manner. Children suffer from different diseases, which may create differences in drug handling. The effects of drugs on growth and development are also important.

It has been suggested that there may be a higher incidence of ADRs when drugs are used in an unlicensed or off-label manner. The evidence is unclear, but it is undoubtedly a major cause for concern. Drugs tested in clinical trials are likely to have ADRs detected at an early stage due to the close monitoring of patient responses. Unlicensed and off-label drugs used in the everyday clinical setting are not monitored to this extent. It follows that ADRs may be missed or observed too late.

Licensed drugs undergo extensive post-marketing surveillance to detect ADRs, which may only become apparent on widespread use. This relies on spontaneous reporting by prescribers, but they may feel inhibited in reporting on the use of unlicensed and off-label drugs. However, regulatory bodies have encouraged such reporting to detect unrecognised interactions and adverse effects. ADR reporting can ultimately be used to reduce the incidence of ADRs, resulting in reduced patient morbidity and mortality.

Medication errors
Medication errors are recognised as an important cause of ADRs in children. The lack of suitable, licensed formulations for children increases the risk of medication errors by complicating administration. For example, a small proportion of the content of an injection vial is frequently required to administer a calculated dose; displacement values must be taken into account and syringes have to be used carefully to avoid administration of the contents of the 'dead space' and overdosing with a concentrated drug.

Extemporaneous dispensing increases the risk of medication errors, since standards of extemporaneous dispensing are extremely variable. Hence, extemporaneous dispensing should be seen as a last resort.

Dosage in children
Children are not 'mini-adults', and doses should not be extrapolated from an adult dose but should be calculated with the help of the *BNF for Children* (BNFC) (BMA & RPSGB, 2009) text. Doses in the BNFC are standardised by weight (and therefore require multiplying by the body weight in kilograms to determine the

child's dose); occasionally, the doses have been standardised by body surface area (in m²). The smaller the child, the greater the care needed to ensure that the dose of drug is correct.

For most drugs, the adult maximum dose should not be exceeded. For example, if the dose is 8 mg/kg with a maximum of 300 mg, a child of 40 kg body weight should receive 300 mg rather than 320 mg. For certain drugs, young children may require a higher dose per kilogram than adults because of a higher metabolic rate. Calculation by body weight in an overweight child may result in much higher doses being administered than necessary; in such cases, the dose should be calculated from an ideal weight related to height and age.

Body surface area estimates (body surface area can be calculated as follows: body surface area (m) = $0.007184 \times$ (patient height in cm)$^{0.725} \times$ (patient weight in kg)$^{0.425}$) are more accurate for calculating paediatric doses than body weight, since many physiological phenomena such as cardiac output, fluid requirements and renal function correlate better with body surface area. In practice, however, using body surface area for dose calculations is only appropriate for a limited number of drugs, such as cytotoxic agents. This is because body surface area can increase by 1–2% per day in a young child and therefore doses require frequent adjustments. Surface area estimations from height/weight nomograms can be problematic because height is difficult to measure accurately, especially in small children. Weight-based nomograms are now available and are used in children's cancer study group protocols within the UK. Only a few published dose recommendations are surface area based, making this method impractical for many drugs.

In selecting a method of dose calculation, the therapeutic index of the drug should be considered. For drugs with a wide therapeutic index, such as penicillin, single doses may be quoted for a wide age range, e.g. 62.5 mg four times daily for children aged 1 month to 1 year. For narrow therapeutic margin index drugs, such as cytotoxic drugs, dosing must be based on calculated surface, with the exception of children under 1 year, where doses of cytotoxic drugs are based on weight to prevent overestimation of the dose in this age group. Between these two extremes comes the dose calculated in milligrams per kilogram. Whichever dose method is used, the result should be modified according to response and whether adverse effects occur.

BNF for Children

The BNFC covers the use of drugs in children of all ages from newborn infants, including those born prematurely, to individuals aged 18 years (BMA & RPSGB, 2009). It is based on information derived from *Medicines for Children* and the BNF, combined with information from other sources such as hospital paediatric formularies, research studies and systematic reviews. It is published annually each July and is also available online (the full content of the BNFC is available without charge at http://bnfc.org or www. bnfc.nhs.uk for those who live in the UK) and digitally.

Whereas the 'standard' BNF deals with the use of medicines for individuals of all ages, the BNFC is able to focus specifically on the use of medicines in children. This allows it to deal with the drug management of childhood conditions more extensively, and it also allows a greater discussion of the unlicensed use of medicines. The BNFC includes advice on drugs used for rare metabolic disorders and on specialist neonatal and paediatric interventions.

Entries on individual drugs give an indication of the licensed status of the drug and if specialist expertise is required for use in children. Recognising that 'adult' conditions may also be relevant to younger individuals, the BNFC includes, in drug entries, advice on the use of medicines during pregnancy and whilst breast-feeding.

The BNFC includes information on drugs when there is sufficient evidence for the drug to be considered relatively safe and effective in children. For some drugs information is very scarce, and their use may be limited to specialist centres and by clinicians with specialist expertise and knowledge of these drugs. In such cases, until the evidence is better established, the BNFC omits information about the drugs.

The use of age bands in the presentation of doses can be confusing. In the BNFC, a dose for, say, 'child 1–8 years' means that the dose may be used from the child's first birthday to the eighth birthday and the next band, say, 'child 8–12 years' applies between a child's eighth and twelfth birthdays. The age bands apply to children of average size, and in practice the clinician will use the age bands in conjunction with other factors such as the severity of the condition being treated and the child's size in relation to the average size of children of the same age.

The BNFC is for use by all health professionals, in all sectors of health care, who are involved in prescribing, administering or managing medicines used for children. The resource is also very well suited to professional training. When used for making clinical decisions, it should be interpreted in the light of professional knowledge and supplemented by specialist literature if necessary. The BNFC is constantly revised so for the latest guidelines the health professional should consult the current edition at BNFC.org.

The BNFC is produced by the BNF Publications editorial team under the supervision of a Paediatric Formulary Committee. A network of expert clinical advisers provides advice and information on current best practice. The names of all individuals who have contributed can be found in the Preface. The BNFC is published under the joint imprint of the British Medical Association, the Royal Pharmaceutical Society of Great Britain, the RCPCH and the NPPG. The BNFC is distributed to all NHS staff and contractors by the Department of Health.

MEDICATION SAFETY IN CHILDREN

Every year over 28 000 children receive treatment for poisoning or suspected poisoning accidents (Consumer Safety Unit, 2002). Medicines are the most common cause of poisoning in children between the ages of 2 and 4 years. Putting a few simple measures in place can stop this happening to children (see www.direct.gov.uk/en/Parents/Yourchildshealthandsafety/Yourchildssafetyinthehome/DG_078861):

- All solid dose and all oral and external liquid preparations should be dispensed in a child-resistant container unless the medicine is in an original pack or patient pack such as to make this inadvisable or no suitable child-resistant container exists for a particular liquid preparation.
- Caps must be kept closed on medicine bottles, and all medicines should be stored away immediately. While child-

resistant caps may slow a child down, they are not child-proof.

- Medicines should be kept well out of reach and out of sight of young children.
- Medicines should be stored in a high cupboard, a cupboard fitted with a child-resistant catch, a lockable cabinet or even a lockable suitcase. Most people keep their medicine cabinet in the bathroom, where it can be hot and steamy, and it could be better placed elsewhere in the home. Medicines should not be kept on a bedside table (a child can easily get into the bedroom without being seen) or in a handbag (this is a favourite place for toddlers to find tablets).
- Some medicines need to be kept in the fridge, but most need to be kept at room temperature, away from direct sunlight and heat sources, such as radiators or fires. The label should give storage instructions but check with your pharmacist if unsure.
- All medicines should be kept in their original containers, so it is clear what is in them and it is harder for children to open them. It can be dangerous to 'decant' medicines into another container as it will be unlabelled, which could be dangerous if different medicines get mixed up and are taken at the wrong time. Some medicines do not work as well once they have be removed from the packaging, such as tablets or capsules that come in blister packs. In addition to showing the name of the medicine, the packaging usually protects it as well.
- Extra care should be taken with tablets in see-through packs or brightly coloured tablets – they are especially tempting to children.
- Parents should be advised to take their medicine when their children are not around so that the children do not try to copy their parents.
- Children should be taught about the safe use of medicines and never pretend that they are sweets.
- Left-over medicines should be taken to the local pharmacy for disposal.
- Parents should be advised to keep an eye on their children in other people's houses, as they may not follow the safety rules above about storing medicines.

Locking medicines away is only the start. It is all too easy for parents to inadvertently overdose their children. US research suggests that 70% of parents have difficulty working out what dose to give their children and that many parents are not aware that combining cold and cough remedies with pain relievers that contain the same active ingredient may result in an overdose. Such an overdose can affect a young child's heart rate and raise their blood pressure, putting them at risk of a stroke. Parents should be advised to follow the tips given below:

- Consult a doctor before giving any over-the-counter medicine to a child under the age of 2 years.
- Never give a child medicine that is designed for adults – even if the parent reduces the dose, it will still be too strong for the child.
- Never give a child a combination of medicines without asking a doctor or pharmacist whether it is safe to do so.
- Read the information leaflet that comes with the medicine in order to learn about any potential side effects before giving medicine to a child.
- Carefully follow the dosage instructions for a child's age and weight. If a child is younger than the recommended age limit stated on the medicine container, then the medicine should not be administered to the child.
- Use the measuring cup or syringe provided to measure out the dose – never 'guesstimate'.
- Never give a child more than the recommended dose, even if he or she is particularly ill.
- Never give a child aspirin, as it has been linked with a rare illness called Reyes syndrome. The government warns that children under the age of 16 years should not be given aspirin unless it is at the direction of a doctor.
- Store medicines (and supplements) safely as described above.
- If an overdose is suspected, take the child to the local A&E immediately, bringing the medicine with them. If the parents have concerns about the dose to give their child, then they should speak to their doctor, pharmacist, NHS Direct on 0845 4647 (England and Wales) or NHS 24 on 08454 24 24 24 (Scotland).

Most children admitted to hospital or seen by GP services are treated safely, but some are exposed to preventable adverse effects. There were 910 089 incidents reported to the National Patient Safety Agency's (NPSA) Reporting and Learning System (RLS) over a 1-year period (1 October 2007 to 30 September 2008) (National Reporting and Learning Service, 2009). Of these, 2% were found to relate to the care of neonates and 5% to the care of children.

The majority of patient safety incidents involving children and neonates were reported to have resulted in no harm or low harm to the child.

'Medication incidents' were the most commonly reported incident type for children (17%), whereas for neonates this was the second most common incident type (15%). Of all medication incidents reported to the RLS (in which an age was provided), nearly 10% involved patients aged between birth and 4 years; this group accounted for the second highest percentage of incidents, similar to that of the oldest groups (those aged 75 years and above).

Administration of the incorrect dose or strength of medication was the highest reported medication incident type for both children and neonates, making up 23% of the overall total of medication incidents for children and 18% for neonates. The second most commonly reported type of medication incident for both children and neonates involved the omission of a medicine or ingredient (10% for children and 18% for neonates). The third most common was the wrong frequency of treatment (8% for children and 13% for neonates).

The finding that dosing errors are the most common type of medication incident for children is consistent with other relevant meta-analyses.

A key contributing factor to dosing errors for children and neonates is the complexity of the dose calculation required. These calculations, based on the age, weight and clinical condition of the child, often require the healthcare professional who is calculating the dose to use only part of a tablet or ampoule intended as an adult preparation. In addition, liquid preparations are often used enterally with younger children when it is not possible to use the oral route. These liquid preparations are available in various strengths, thereby increasing the possibility of a dosing incident.

Some children's medicines require the healthcare professional to convert dose units from milligrams to micrograms due to the availability of drug preparations. This results in calculations involving decimal points, which have been considered a factor in the occurrence of 10-fold dosing errors within a child's and neo-natal environment, e.g. diamorphine and morphine injections – the lowest strengths of licensed diamorphine and morphine injections are 5 mg and 10 mg, respectively; one such ampoule is sufficient to cause an overdose of 10 or 100 times in neonates.

Other examples of commonly used drugs in paediatric and neonatal medicine where 10-fold overdoses have occurred are benzylpenicillin, theophylline, digoxin, tacrolimus, adrenaline and cyclosporin.

The number of medication incidents involving IV medication preparation and administration is large. A multicentre audit concluded that the incidence of medication errors with IV medication preparation and administration is higher than with other forms of medicine. For example, gentamicin is an antibiotic widely used intravenously for the treatment of neonatal sepsis. It has a narrow therapeutic range; high trough concentrations may cause oto- and/or nephrotoxicity, and low peak levels will affect efficacy. An analysis search of RLS data undertaken for the period April 2007 to March 2008 for neonatal medication incident involving gentamicin found 400 relevant incidents. Of these, 66% were related to problems with administration, 23% with prescribing and 6% with monitoring.

Gentamicin is the subject of a joint project between the NPSA and the RCPCH, the 'Safer Practice in Neonatal Care – care bundle' project. Care bundles are defined as 'a group of evidence-based interventions related to a disease or care process that, when executed together, result in better outcomes than when implemented individually.' One of the two care bundles piloted across neonatal units in England is related to the safe administration of IV gentamicin to neonates. Elements of this care bundle include:

- a policy of no interruptions during the prescribing, preparing, checking and administering process;

- the use of the 24-h clock when prescribing;
- administration of the dose to be given within 1 h either side of the prescribed time;
- a prompt checklist for nurses administering the drug.

CONCLUSION
This chapter has provided an overview of medications management in children. The factors affecting drug disposition in children have been discussed and the principles of prescribing in children have been outlined. Medication safety in children has been described.

REFERENCES
British Medical Association, Royal Pharmaceutical Society of Great Britain, Royal College of Paediatrics and Child Health and Neonatal and Paediatric Pharmacists Group (2009) *BNF for Children* (BNFC). BMJ Publishing Group Ltd, RPS Publishing, RCPCH Publications Ltd, London.

Conroy S (2003) Paediatric pharmacy-drug therapy. *Hosp Pharm* **10**: 49–57.

Consumer Safety Unit (2002) *24th Annual Report, Home Accident Surveillance System*. Department of Trade and Industry, London.

Morkane C, Binns K, Coleman J (2007) The medic's guide to prescribing: prescribing for children. *Student BMJ* **15**: 293–336.

National Prescribing Centre (2000) Prescribing for children MeReC Bulletin Volume 11 Number 2. Liverpool. Available at www.npc.co.uk/ebt/merec/other_non_clinical/resources/merec_bulletin_vol11_no2.pdf

National Reporting and Learning Service (2009) *Review of Patient Safety for Children and Young People*. Available at www.npsa.nhs.uk/nrls.

National Service Framework for Children, Young People and Maternity Services (2004) *Medicines for Children and Young People*. Department of Health, London.

Nursing & Midwifery Council (NMC) (2007) *Standards for Medicines Management*. NMC, London. Available at http://www.nmc-uk.org/aDisplayDocument.aspx?DocumentID=6978.

Scottish Neonatal and Paediatric Pharmacists Group (SNAPP), NHS Education for Scotland (NES) *Introduction to Paediatric Pharmaceutical Care*. Available at www.nppg.org.uk.

14 | Nurse Prescribing

Elizabeth Payne

INTRODUCTION

Nurse prescribing in the UK was first advocated in the 1986 Cumberlege Report (*Neighbourhood Nursing: A focus for care*) (Department of Health and Social Security, 1986). It recommended that community nurses should be able to prescribe from a limited list of items agreed by the Department of Health.

In 1989, a Department of Health Advisory Group chaired by Dr June Crown, Director of Public Health, considered the implications that nurse prescribing raised and published the first Crown Report [Department of Health (DH), 1989], which recommended that suitably qualified registered nurses (defined as those with a district nurse or health visitor qualification) should be authorised to prescribe from a limited list, the Nurse Prescribers' Formulary, and adjust the timing and dosage of medicines within a set protocol.

Primary legislation permitting nurses to prescribe was passed in 1992. This was the Medicinal Products: Prescription by Nurses and Others Act 1992. Chapter 28, Article 1(d) of this act defines a nurse prescriber as 'any registered nurse, midwife or health visitor'. Between 1994 and 1998 pilot sites were established, and in 1998 a national roll-out of nurse prescribing was announced and the first limited national formulary was published – now called the *Nurse Prescribers' Formulary for Community Practitioners*. This programme of nurse prescribing, which was completed in spring 2001, applied only to nurses with district nurse or health visitor qualifications.

In order to become a community practitioner prescriber, health visitors and district nurses were required to complete a distance learning package and 3-day training course (at an approved higher education institute) assessed by written examination.

In 1999, another advisory group, again chaired by Dr June Crown, reviewed more widely the prescribing, supply and administration of medicines. It recommended (in the second Crown Report) (DH, 1999) the establishing of two groups of nurse prescribers, independent and supplementary, as well as extending prescribing rights to nurses, pharmacists, physiotherapists, chiropodists/podiatrists and optometrists. (It was not until 2005 that the healthcare professionals listed, with the exception of nurses and pharmacists, were granted supplementary prescribing rights).

In 2000, the NHS plan endorsed this recommendation. In May 2001, the government announced that 'independent' prescribing responsibilities would be extended to enable more groups of nurses to prescribe a wider range of medicines (the Health and Social Care Act 2001), and by 2002 the Nurse Prescribers Extended Formulary (NPEF) (DH, 2004) was introduced for four therapeutic areas: minor injuries, minor ailments, health promotion and palliative care. The Nursing & Midwifery Council (NMC) introduced the first 'independent' or extended formulary nurse prescriber course.

Finally, in November 2002 nurses and pharmacists were granted the right to prescribe medicines, not only as extended formulary prescribers but also as supplementary prescribers, or supply medicines under patient group directions, previously known as group protocols. In 2004, the NMC changed the nurse prescriber course to a dual 'independent'/supplementary prescriber course.

Work to expand the NPEF took place from 2003 to 2005. By May 2005, the NPEF included around 240 prescription-only medicines (POMs), together with all pharmacy (P) and general sales list (GSL) medicines prescribable by GPs for defined medical conditions. Consultation on the options for future-independent prescribing by nurses took place in early 2005. This led to recommendations in November 2005 and the subsequent introduction of nurse independent prescribers.

From May 2006, nurses who were nurse independent prescribers (formally known as extended formulary prescribers) could, with the exception of some controlled drugs, prescribe medicines from the *British National Formulary* for any medical condition, replacing the need for the NPEF (DH, 2006). Nurse independent prescribers could also prescribe from the *BNF for Children* (BNFC), where appropriate.

The aim of this chapter is to provide an overview to nurse prescribing.

LEARNING OUTCOMES
At the end of this chapter, the reader will be able to:

❑ Define nurse prescribing.
❑ List the nurse practitioners who can prescribe.
❑ Discuss what can be prescribed by nurse prescribers.
❑ Outline best practice for nurse prescribing.
❑ Discuss the principles of nurse prescribing.

DEFINITION OF NURSE PRESCRIBING
A prescriber is a qualified professional who has undergone formal theoretical and practical training as part of an accredited programme of study and has been assessed as being competent and confident to prescribe.

The nurses' titles given in Table 14.1 and recorded on the NMC Register reflect the changes to nurse prescribing rights and definitions that took effect from 1 May 2006 subsequent to the amendments in prescribing legislation. V100, V200 and V300 refer to Department of Health-approved training courses.

Table 14.1 Previous and currently recognised nurse prescriber titles

Previous definition	Current definition
District nurse/health visitor formulary nurses and any nurse undertaking the V100 prescribing programme as part of a Specialist Practitioner qualification	Community practitioner nurse prescribers (V100) Able to prescribe from the nurse formulary in the current month's Drug Tariff (www.ppa.org.uk/edt/January_2010/mindex.htm; see Electronic Drug Tariff) and in the BNF
Extended formulary nurse prescribers	Nurse independent prescribers (V200) only
Extended/supplementary nurse prescribers	Nurse independent/supplementary prescribers (V300)

NURSE PRACTITIONERS WHO CAN PRESCRIBE

Community practitioner nurse prescribers

Community practitioner nurse prescribers who have successfully completed the V100 prescribing course may prescribe from a limited formulary of products, containing 13 POMs, some P and GSL medicines, and a list of dressings and appliances relevant to community nursing and health visiting practice, found in the Nurse Prescribers' Formulary for Community Practitioners in the *British National Formulary* (BNF) (British Medical Association and Royal Pharmaceutical Society of Great Britain, 2009) and Part XV11B(i) of the Drug Tariff (Drug Tariff available online at www.ppa.org.uk/edt/January_2010/mindex.htm).

Nurse independent prescribers

Nurse independent prescribers are those who have successfully completed the V300 prescribing course. They may prescribe either as independent prescribers or as supplementary prescribers.

They *must only* prescribe medications for patients if it is appropriate to the individual prescriber's level of expertise, it is within their scope of professional practice and they are clinically competent and confident to do so.

Nurse independent prescribing is not suitable for prescribing for complex medical conditions or for patients with several co-morbidities.

Nurse supplementary prescribers

Supplementary prescribing is a voluntary partnership between the medical/dental prescriber and a supplementary prescriber, to implement an agreed patient-specific clinical management plan (CMP) with the patient's agreement. Supplementary prescribers should only enter into a prescribing partnership that requires them to prescribe medication they feel competent to prescribe.

Nurse supplementary prescribers with a V300 qualification may prescribe medication that has been initiated by a medical/dental prescriber for patients with long-term medical conditions or with long-term health needs. The patient must agree to the nurse taking on this responsibility, and the CMP must specify the changes the nurse supplementary prescriber can make to the patient's medication and under what circumstances a referral to the medical prescriber is necessary.

Supplementary prescribing is not suited to emergency, urgent or acute prescribing situations because an agreed CMP is needed before prescribing can begin.

WHAT CAN BE PRESCRIBED BY NURSE PRESCRIBERS

Community practitioner nurse prescribers

Community practitioner nurse prescribers may only prescribe the dressings, appliances and licensed medicines listed in the Nurse Prescribers' Formulary for Community Practitioners. The one exception to this is the prescription of nystatin off label for neonates for oral thrush at the dose recommended in the BNFC. This exception is allowed on the basis that there is no systemic absorption of nystatin and the use of the product in treatment of oral thrush is long established.

Nurse independent prescribers

Nurse independent prescribers have, with the exception of some controlled drugs, unrestricted prescribing rights for any licensed medicine in the BNF, a list of which can be found in the monthly Drug Tariff (see part XVIIB(ii)). Nurse independent prescribers are expected to take into account the local formulary policies of their employing organisation and the implications for primary care.

Nurse independent prescribers can prescribe the controlled drugs listed in Table 14.2 solely for the specified routes and medical conditions. Only nurse independent prescribers have the authority to do this; no other non-medical prescriber can prescribe controlled drugs.

Proposed changes to Home Office Misuse of Drugs Regulations mean that these restrictions may be removed in the near future. If approved, nurse and pharmacist independent prescribers will be able to independently prescribe any schedule 2, 3, 4 and 5 controlled drug. [Schedule 1 controlled drugs include the hallucinogenic drugs (for example LSD) and ecstasy-type substances, which have virtually no therapeutic use].

Table 14.2 Controlled drugs prescribable by Nurse Independent Prescribers solely for the medical conditions indicated

Substance	Route of administration	Specified medical condition
Buprenorphine	Transdermal	Palliative care
Chlordiazepoxide	Oral	Treatment of initial or acute withdrawal symptoms, caused by the withdrawal of alcohol from persons habituated to it
Diamorphine hydrochloride	Oral or parenteral	Suspected myocardial infarction or for relief of acute or severe pain after trauma, including in either case post-operative pain relief Palliative care
Fentanyl	Transdermal	Palliative care
Morphine sulphate	Oral, parenteral or rectal	Suspected myocardial infarction or for relief of acute or severe pain after trauma, including in either case post-operative pain relief Palliative care
Morphine hydrochloride	Rectal	Suspected myocardial infarction or for relief of acute or severe pain after trauma, including in either case post-operative pain relief Palliative care
Oxycodone hydrochloride	Oral or parenteral administration in palliative care	Palliative care
Diazepam	Oral, parenteral or rectal	Tonic-clonic seizures Treatment of initial or acute withdrawal symptoms, caused by the withdrawal of alcohol from persons habituated to it Palliative care
Lorazepam	Oral or parenteral	Tonic-clonic seizures Palliative care
Midazolam	Parenteral or buccal	Tonic-clonic seizures Palliative care
Codeine phosphate	Oral	–
Dihydrocodeine tartrate	Oral	–
Co-phenotrope	Oral	–

Nurse independent prescribers can prescribe borderline substances, but the Department of Health recommends that they restrict their prescribing to the substances on the Advisory Committee on Borderline Substances approved list, in Part XV of the Drug Tariff.

Nurse independent prescribers can prescribe medicines off label where it is best practice to do so or there are clinical trials demonstrating the use and safety of the medicine for that clinical indication.

Until recently, nurse independent prescribers have not been authorised to prescribe unlicensed medicines. However, as a result of extensive consultation by the MHRA from December 2008 onwards, legislation [see The Medicines for Human Use (Miscellaneous Amendments) (No.2) Regulations 2009 SI 3062: www.opsi.gov.uk/si/si2009/uksi_20093062_en_1] has been amended, and came into force on 21 December 2009, to allow nurse and pharmacist independent prescribers to prescribe unlicensed medicines in all clinical areas, for use by his/her individual patient on his/her personal responsibility (RPSGB, 2009). This includes prescribing a mixture of two licensed drugs for administration (where one is not the vehicle for administration of the other), for example via a syringe drive in palliative care, since this creates an unlicensed drug.

The NMC (NMC, 2006) and the Royal Pharmaceutical Society of Great Britain (RPSGB, 2007) advise that nurse independent prescribers should not prescribe any medicine for themselves. Independent nurse prescribers are accountable for their practice at all times, and if a situation arises where they find themselves in a position to prescribe for their family or friends, then they must accept accountability for that decision. It is strongly recommended that nurse independent prescribers do not prescribe for anyone with whom they have a close personal or emotional relationship other than in exceptional circumstances.

Supplementary prescribers

Supplementary nurse prescribers can prescribe any medicine that is referred to in a patient's CMP agreed by a medical/dental prescriber.

The CMP (written or electronic) must:

- be in place before supplementary prescribing can occur;
- be specific to a named patient/client and to that patient/client's specific condition(s) to be managed by the supplementary prescriber;
- include details of the illness or conditions that may be treated, the class or description of medical products that can be prescribed or administered, and the circumstances in which the supplementary prescriber should refer to, or seek advice from, the medical prescriber.

An example of a CMP template is available on www.nelm. nhs.uk/en/NeLM-Area/Community-Areas/Non-Medical-Prescribing/Support-Materials/ and www.cmponline.info/.

There are no legal restrictions on the clinical conditions that supplementary nurse prescribers may treat. However, it is for the medical/dental prescriber with the supplementary nurse prescriber to decide, in drawing up the CMP, when supplementary prescribing is appropriate.

Provided medicines are prescribable by the medical/dental prescriber at NHS expense, and they are referred to in the patient's CMP, supplementary nurse prescribers are able to prescribe, at NHS expense, the following:

- all GSL medicines, P medicines, appliances and devices, foods, and other borderline substances approved by the Advisory Committee on Borderline Substances;
- all POMs and controlled drugs except those listed in Schedule 1 to the Misuse of Drug Regulations 2001, which are not intended for medicinal use;
- off-label medicines, black triangle drugs and drugs marked 'less suitable for prescribing' in the BNF;
- unlicensed medicines.

BEST PRACTICE FOR NURSE PRESCRIBING

The Standards of Proficiency for Nurse and Midwife Prescribers (NMC, 2006) provide the standards of conduct that nurses, midwives and specialist community public health nurses are required to meet in their practice as registered nurse prescribers.

Nurse prescribers must have sufficient knowledge and competence to be able to:

- assess a patient/client's clinical condition;
- undertake a thorough history, including medical history and medication history, and diagnose where necessary;
- decide on how to manage the condition and whether it is necessary to prescribe or not;
- identify appropriate medication if required;
- advise the patient/client/client on the benefits and risks of treatment;
- prescribe if the patient/client agrees;
- monitor the response to medication;
- provide lifestyle advice where appropriate.

The standards for prescribing practice, described below, apply to *all* settings, in which a registrant may prescribe, within the NHS, independent sector, armed forces or prison service.

Practice standard 1: Licence as a prescriber

In order to practise as a nurse prescriber, a nurse must first successfully complete an NMC-approved prescribing programme, which is recorded in the NMC Register. Once licensed, nurse prescribers may only prescribe from the formulary linked to their recorded qualification and must comply with statutory requirements applicable to their prescribing practice, as well as with any local policies drawn up by their employer.

Practice standard 2: Accountability

Nurse prescribers are professionally accountable for their prescribing decisions, including actions and omissions, and cannot delegate this accountability to any other person. A nurse prescriber must only ever prescribe within their level of experience and competence, especially when moving to another area of practice or new role, in accordance with Clause 6 of *The NMC Code of Professional Conduct: Standards for Conduct, Performance and Ethics* (NMC, 2008).

In a situation where a nurse prescriber is expected to assess and prescribe outside their 'normal' field of practice, they must refer the patient/client to an appropriate prescriber, even though they may be able to take a thorough and appropriate history that leads to a diagnosis.

Practice standard 3: Assessment

A nurse prescriber must be satisfied that they have fully assessed the patient/client; this includes taking a thorough history and, where possible, accessing a full clinical record. This is essential since a nurse prescriber must only prescribe where they have relevant knowledge of the patient/client's health and medical history, and where they have undertaken a risk assessment of the patient/client's current medication and any potential for confusion with other medicines.

Practice standard 4: Need

A nurse prescriber must only prescribe where there is a genuine clinical need for treatment.

Practice standard 5: Consent

A nurse prescriber must obtain the patient/client's consent before prescribing in accordance with Clause 3 of *The NMC Code of Professional Conduct: Standards for Conduct, Performance and Ethics* (NMC, 2008).

A nurse prescriber must make it clear to the patient/client that prescribing cannot be undertaken in isolation. The nurse prescriber must inform, where relevant, anyone else who may be in a position to prescribe for that patient/client, such as the patient/ client's general/medical practitioner or other independent/ supplementary prescriber looking after the patient/client, of their actions in order to avoid prescribing errors.

Practice standard 6: Communication

A nurse prescriber must communicate effectively with other practitioners involved in the care of the patient/client and refer the patient/client to another prescriber where appropriate.

Practice standard 7: Record keeping

A nurse prescriber is responsible for keeping accurate, comprehensive, up-to-date records that record the details of the patient/ client consultation, as well as prescription details, and are accessible by all members of a prescribing team, in accordance with local policies. The same common patient/client record must be consulted and used by the medical/dental prescriber and supplementary nurse prescriber wherever possible. The NMC *Guidelines for records and record keeping* (NMC, 2009) provide the underlying principles.

The maximum time between writing a prescription and recording the details should not exceed 48 h.

Practice standard 8: Clinical management plans (supplementary prescribing)

A nurse supplementary prescriber must prescribe according to a patient/client's individual CMP, or a standard CMP that has been modified to reflect the individual patient/client's personal, medical and medicines history. The medical/dental prescriber must have made the initial diagnosis of the patient/client.

The CMP must be agreed by a medical/dental prescriber and the nurse prescriber, with the agreement and consent of the patient/client, before supplementary prescribing begins. Confirmation of agreement may be in the form of a signature or, for an electronic record, a recordable indication of agreement. Alternatively, the medical/dental prescriber may agree verbally to a CMP provided that it is confirmed by fax or secure e-mail before prescribing occurs and formally agreed within 2 working days.

A nurse supplementary prescriber must *never* prescribe medication without a CMP and must refer the patient/client back to the doctor/dentist when the patient/clients' circumstances fall outside the CMP. It is a criminal offence for a nurse supplementary prescriber to prescribe a POM outside a CMP, and in the case of a non-POM, the nurse prescriber would be subject to disciplinary proceedings by their employer and referral to the NMC for misconduct.

Practice standard 9: Prescribing and administration/supply

A nurse prescriber must ensure that the activities of prescribing and administration of medicines are kept separate. However, in exceptional circumstances, where the nurse prescriber is involved in both prescribing and administering a patient/client's controlled drug, a second suitably competent person should be involved in checking the accuracy of the medication provided.

Practice standard 10: Prescribing and dispensing

A nurse prescriber must ensure that the activities of prescribing and dispensing are kept separate, whenever possible. However, in exceptional circumstances, where the nurse prescriber is involved in both prescribing and dispensing a patient/client's medication, a second suitably competent person should be involved in checking the accuracy of the medication provided. The nurse prescriber should obtain indemnity insurance to cover any dispensing that may occur. *Note*: Dispensing is defined as the 'labelling' of medication from a stock supply that is then administered to a patient/client.

Practice standard 11: Prescribing for family and others (excluding controlled drugs – see Practice standard 16)

Nurse prescribers must not prescribe for themselves or for anyone with whom they have a close personal or emotional relationship, other than in an exceptional circumstance. If a prescription is necessary, the nurse prescriber should refer this to be undertaken by another registered prescriber wherever possible.

Practice standard 12: Computer-generated prescribing by nurses or midwives

A nurse prescriber can use appropriate software to prescribe via computer-generated prescription but must keep a visible audit trail of prescribing actions.

Nurse prescribers must never tamper with existing prescriber's details on a prescription or add their own prescribing details, whether that be handwritten or by stamp.

Prescriptions should always be signed immediately, never written/printed off and signed in advance and then stored for future use.

Practice standard 13: Evidence-based prescribing

A nurse prescriber should be aware of, and apply, local and national prescribing guidelines so their prescribing practice is evidence based. The nurse prescriber should be familiar with current guidance in the BNF. Where local guidelines differ from national guidelines, the nurse prescriber should obtain guidance through their employer's clinical governance structure.

Practice standard 14: Delegation
Nurse prescribers may delegate the administration of a medication that they have prescribed but must be satisfied that the person who is to administer the medication is suitably trained and competent to do so.

Practice standard 15: Continuing professional development
Nurse prescribers are responsible for keeping their knowledge and skills up to date, and ensuring that their continuing professional development reflects their role as prescribers, in accordance with Clause 6 of *The NMC Code of Professional Conduct: Standards for Conduct, Performance and Ethics* (NMC, 2008).

Practice standard 16: Controlled drugs
Prescribing controlled drugs
A nurse prescriber must only prescribe controlled drugs that they are legally entitled to prescribe, in accordance with legal prescribing requirements (summarised in the BNF). The nurse prescriber must ensure that the patient/client's NHS number or other patient/client-specific indicator is included in the prescription form, the dosage instructions are specified to avoid uncertainty on administration (care with syringe driver prescriptions), the quantity of any controlled drug prescribed (excluding those in schedule 5) does not exceed 28 days' supply per prescription except in exceptional circumstances and is endorsed appropriately by the nurse prescriber, and the registration number of the prescriber is included on the prescription.

The nurse prescriber may use computer-generated prescriptions for all controlled drugs, as specified under Practice standard 12, but must ensure that the most up-to-date documentation is used.

The nurse prescriber must inform anyone who needs to know about any restrictions placed on their prescribing practice, particularly pharmacists with dispensing responsibilities.

Prescribing controlled drugs for oneself
A nurse prescriber must *not* prescribe a controlled drug for themselves.

Prescribing controlled drugs for someone close
A nurse prescriber may only prescribe a controlled drug for someone close to them if:

- no other person with the legal right to prescribe is available;
- and then only if that treatment is immediately necessary to:
  ○ save life;
  ○ avoid significant deterioration in the patient/client's health;
  ○ alleviate otherwise uncontrollable pain.

Nurse prescribers must be able to justify their actions and must document their relationship and the emergency circumstances that necessitated prescribing a controlled drug for someone close to them.

Practice standard 17: Prescribing unlicensed medicines
A nurse prescriber may prescribe an unlicensed medication both as an independent prescriber or as a supplementary prescriber as part of a CMP providing:

- the medical/dental prescriber and the nurse prescriber, acting as a supplementary prescriber, have agreed the plan with the patient/client in a voluntary relationship;
- the nurse prescriber is satisfied that an alternative, licensed medication would not meet the patient/client's needs;
- the nurse prescriber is satisfied that there is a sufficient evidence base and/or experience to demonstrate the medication's safety and efficacy for that particular patient/client;
- the medical/dental prescriber is prepared to take the responsibility for prescribing the unlicensed medicine and has agreed the patient/client's CMP to that effect;
- the patient/client agrees to a prescription in the knowledge that the drug is unlicensed and understands the implications of this;
- the medication chosen and the reason for choosing it are documented in the CMP.

Practice standard 18: Prescribing medicines for use outside the terms of their licence (off-label)

A nurse independent prescriber may prescribe off-label or licensed medicines for the purposes for which they are not licensed under the following circumstances:

- It would better serve the patient/client's needs to have an off-label medicine than an appropriately licensed alternative.
- There is a sufficient evidence base and/or experience of using the medicine to demonstrate its safety and efficacy.
- The nurse prescriber has explained to the patient/client, or parent/carer, in broad terms, the reasons why medicines are not licensed for their proposed use.
- The nurse prescriber has made a clear, accurate and legible record of all medicines prescribed and the reasons for prescribing an off-label medicine.

A nurse supplementary prescriber may prescribe off label providing:

- there is a CMP in place, written in conjunction with the medical/dental prescriber and in voluntary partnership with the patient/client or parent/carer;
- a medical/dental prescriber takes responsibility for prescribing the medicine, and the nurse prescriber jointly oversees the patient/client's care, monitors the patient and ensures that any follow-up treatment is given as required.

Practice standard 19: Repeat prescribing

A nurse prescriber may issue a repeat prescription, but must be satisfied that it is safe and appropriate to do so and that secure procedures are in place to ensure that:

- the patient/client is issued with the correct prescription;
- each prescription is regularly reviewed and is only re-issued to meet clinical need;
- a review takes place following a maximum of six prescriptions or 6 months elapsing;
- the correct dose is prescribed;
- suitable provision is in place to monitor each patient/client's condition and ensure that patient/clients who need a further

examination or assessment do not receive repeat prescriptions without being seen by an appropriate prescriber.

Practice standard 20: Remote prescribing via telephone, e-mail, fax, video link or website

It may be appropriate, on occasion, to use a telephone or other non face-to-face medium to prescribe medicines and treatment for patient/clients. Such situations may occur where:

- the nurse prescriber has responsibility for the care of the patient/client;
- the nurse prescriber is working in remote and rural areas;
- the nurse prescriber has prior knowledge and understanding of the patient/client's condition and medical history;
- the nurse prescriber has authority to access the patient/client's records and is working within the scope of a supplementary prescriber, but the medical/dental prescriber required to authorise the CMP works at a distance.

In all circumstances, the nurse prescriber must ensure that they:

- establish the patient/client's current medical conditions, history, and concurrent or recent use of other medications, including non-prescription medicines;
- carry out an adequate assessment of the patient/client's condition (in line with Practice standard 3);
- identify the likely cause of the patient/client's condition;
- ensure that there is sufficient justification to prescribe the medicines or treatment proposed – where appropriate, the nurse prescriber should discuss other treatment options with the patient/client;
- ensure that the treatment and/or medicine is not contraindicated for the patient/client;
- make a clear, accurate, legible and contemporaneous record of all medicines prescribed;
- are competent to make a prescribing decision.

Where the nurse prescriber cannot meet *all* of these requirements they must *not* use remote means to prescribe medicine for a patient/client.

Practice standard 21: Gifts and benefits

A nurse prescriber must make their choice of medicinal product for the patient/client based on clinical suitability and cost effectiveness, not in response to any inducements. It is an offence to solicit or accept a gift or inducement, and any hospitality for a professional/scientific meeting must be reasonable in level to the purpose of the meeting.

The nurse prescriber must maintain a 'register of interests', in accordance with local corporate policy, within their personal portfolio, which may be produced on request if required for audit purposes.

PRINCIPLES OF NURSE PRESCRIBING

The National Prescribing Centre has outlined seven principles of good prescribing to aid nurse prescribers in their decision making (NPC, 1999). The prescribing process is often complex, and therefore it is important to consider all relevant factors before deciding to prescribe:

- *Consider the patient's needs – is a prescription necessary?*
  Take the patient's medical and social history. It may be useful to use the mnemonic 2-WHAM:

  W – Who is it for?
  W – What are the symptoms?
  H – How long have the symptoms been present?
  A – Any action taken so far?
  M – any other Medication? Check for any over-the-counter medication and complementary therapies such as herbal or homeopathic remedies.

  Identify any drug allergies and record this in the patient's notes.
- *Consider the appropriate strategy*
  Consider whether there is an established diagnosis, whether a GP referral is indicated, whether a prescription is needed at all and whether there is pressure to prescribe as a result of patient expectation.

Consider all treatment options, including non-drug therapy, which may be indicated instead of or complementary to a prescription.

A prescription should only be given where there is a genuine need. Patients may wish to obtain a prescription for reasons other than to gain treatment of their complaint, such as to legitimise the sick role, to gain attention or to get a prescription for a family member or friend.

- *If a prescription is indicated, consider the choice of product*
The use of the mnemonic EASE may help:

E – how Effective is the product?
A – is it Appropriate for this patient?
S – how Safe is it?
E – is the prescription cost-Effective?

The available evidence should be critically appraised in order to assess how effective a product is. The sources of information that may help with this are the BNF, local and national guidelines, and policies such as NICE/MHRA/NPSA/DoH guidance, local prescribing advisors, GPs, community pharmacists, medicine information services (the nearest regional medicines information centre, listed on the inside cover of the BNF, will be able to give a local centre as appropriate) and independent evaluated information such as *MeReC Bulletins and Briefings*, Cochrane Library, *Drug and Therapeutics Bulletin*, Bandolier and so on.

To assess whether a product is appropriate for a patient, it is necessary to refer to the contraindications and cautions section in the BNF or the relevant summary of product characteristics (available under www.emc.medicines.org.uk). The patient's medication history may also reveal potential drug interactions, which may have serious consequences, e.g. the use of simvastatin and HIV protease inhibitors increases the risk of myopathy/rhabdomyolysis. Similarly, this information may be found in the aforementioned sources.

The dose, formulation and duration of treatment should be tailored to individual needs. Particular caution is necessary when prescribing for certain patient groups such as pregnant or breastfeeding women, those at the extremes of age, those with renal or hepatic impairment, and those who may not metabolise and excrete drugs in the way a young or healthy adult does. In pregnant or breastfeeding women, certain drugs may be harmful to the foetus or are excreted in breast milk, causing adverse reactions (ADRs) in the infant. In the other patient groups mentioned, drug clearance may be affected and as a result the risk of toxicity may be higher.

The potential benefits of the treatment must always be balanced against safety concerns; the nurse prescriber should check for any adverse effects reported previous to drug therapy. The nurse prescriber should be familiar with the common adverse drug reactions of the treatment they are prescribing. In order to avoid adverse drug reactions, the patient's drug therapy should be rationalised to include as few drugs as possible with the lowest effective doses. If an ADR occurs, the nurse prescriber should document the details of the reaction in the patient/client's record and inform the patient/client's medical/dental prescriber as appropriate. Furthermore, the ADR should be reported directly to the MHRA through the yellow card scheme, especially if it is a serious reaction to an established drug, a black triangle drug, a vaccine, a medical device or a medicine used in a child.

The nurse prescriber should be aware of the relative costs of treatment in order to make optimum use of the NHS budget once an appropriate course of treatment has been selected. The nurse prescriber should use the generic name of the product when prescribing except in the case of narrow therapeutic drugs, e.g. carbamazepine, theophylline, lithium, as well as dressings and appliances. Prescribing a drug by its generic name is recognised as good prescribing practice and has led to major cost savings. Sometimes, when prescribing a P-only or over-the-counter product, it may be more appropriate to recommend that a patient who is liable to pay prescription charges buys the product from a pharmacy. An annual list of prescribable products, which are cheaper when purchased from a pharmacy is available from Dept DTB, Consumers Association, Castlemead, Gascoyne Way, Hertford X and SG14 1SH (ref OTC98).

- *Negotiate a contract*

  A prescribing decision may be viewed as a shared contract between patient and prescriber. This shared decision making is known as concordance. Concordance values the patient's perspective, acknowledging that the patient has expertise in his or her body's experience of illness and response to treatment. This expertise is different from the professional's scientific expertise in drug treatment selection but is of equal relevance and value in terms of deciding on best management. A concordant consultation is one that includes both these views in the decision-making process regarding management. A systematic review of the literature relevant to concordance found that two-way communication between patients and professionals about medicines led to improved satisfaction with care, knowledge of the condition and treatment, adherence, health outcomes and fewer medication-related problems.

  Effective communication is an essential part of good practice, as discussed in the *NMC Code of Professional Conduct: Standards for Conduct, Performance and Ethics* (NMC, 2008). This includes the need to ensure that the patients understand relevant information about their treatment such as what the prescription is for, how long it takes to work, how to take the drug, how long to take the drug for, what dose to take, and the possible adverse effects and what to do about these if they occur.

- *Reviewing the patient*

  The patient should be reassessed at least every 6 months, with no more than six repeat prescriptions given without review. Regular review is important to establish whether the treatment prescribed is effective, safe and acceptable; it also reduces the waste of unwanted medication.

- *Keeping records*

  The *NMC guidance for nurses and midwives on recordkeeping* (NMC, 2009) makes it clear that nurses have a professional responsibility to keep accurate and up-to-date records. Details of any treatment prescribed should be recorded in the patient's notes immediately.

- *Reflecting on prescribing*

  The NMC Code of Professional Conduct: Standards for Conduct, Performance and Ethics (NMC, 2008) makes it clear that it is essential for nurses to maintain and improve their professional knowledge and competence. Reviewing and reflecting on prescribing decisions will help nurses to improve their prescribing knowledge and practice. This forms an important part of the nurse prescriber's CPD.

CONCLUSION

This chapter has provided an overview of nurse prescribing. The term 'nurse prescribing' has been defined. The various nurse practitioners who can prescribe have been listed, together with what they can prescribe. Best practice for nurse prescribing has been outlined, and the principles of nurse prescribing have been discussed.

REFERENCES

British Medical Association and Royal Pharmaceutical Society of Great Britain (2009) *British National Formulary*. BMJ Group & RPS Publishing, London. Available at bnf.org/bnf/.

Department of Health and Social Security (1986) Cumberlege Report. *Neighbourhood Nursing: a Focus for Care*. HMSO, London.

Department of Health (1989) Crown Report. *Report of the Advisory Group on Nurse Prescribing*. Department of Health, London.

Department of Health (1999) Crown Report. *Final Report of the Review of Prescribing, Supply and Administration of Medicines*. Department of Health, London.

Department of Health (2004) *Extending Independent Nurse Prescribing within the NHS in England: a Guide for Implementation*, 2nd edn. Department of Health, London. Available at www.dh.gov.uk/dr_consum_dh/groups/dh_digitalassets/@dh/@en/documents/digitalasset/dh_4072177.pdf.

Department of Health (2006) *Improving Patients' Access to Medicines: Implementing Nurse and Pharmacist Prescribing within the NHS in England*: Department of Health, Leeds. Available at www.dh.gov.uk/dr_consum_dh/groups/dh_digitalassets/@dh/@en/documents/digitalasset/dh_4133747.pdf.

Electronic Drug Tariff. Available at www.ppa.org.uk/edt/January_2010/mindex.htm.

MHRA (2007) Public Consultation-Independent Prescribing of Controlled Drugs by Nurse and Pharmacist Independent Prescribers (MLX 338), MHRA. Available at www.mhra.gov.uk/Publications/Consultations/Medicinesconsultations/MLXs/CON2030628.

MHRA (Dec. 2008; July 2009) Public consultation-Proposal (MLX 356) and outcome of consultation exercise on proposals for amendments to medicines legislation to allow mixing of medicines in palliative care. MHRA. Available at www.mhra.gov.uk/Publications/Consultations/Medicinesconsultations/MLXs/CON033523.

National Prescribing Centre (1999) Signposts for prescribing nurses – general principles of good prescribing. *Prescribing Bulletin* **1**, No. 1. Available at www.npc.co.uk/prescribers/resources/nurse_bulletin_vol1no1.pdf.

Nursing & Midwifery Council (2006) *Standards of Proficiency for Nurse and Midwife Prescribers.* NMC, London. Available at www.nmc-uk.org/aDisplayDocument.aspx?documentID=6942.

Nursing & Midwifery Council (2008) *The Code: Standards of Conduct, Performance and Ethics for Nurses and Midwives.* NMC, London. Available at www.nmc-uk.org/aDisplayDocument.aspx?document ID=5982.

Nursing & Midwifery Council (2009) *Record Keeping: Guidance for Nurses and Midwives.* NMC, London. Available at www.nmc-uk.org/aDisplayDocument.aspx?DocumentID=6269.

Royal Pharmaceutical Society of Great Britain (2007) *Professional Standards and Guidance for Pharmacist Prescribers.* RPSGB, London. Available at www.rpsgb.org/pdfs/coepsgpharmpresc.pdf.

Royal Pharmaceutical Society of Great Britain (2009) Law and Ethics Bulletin, 7 December 2009. *Prescribing of Unlicensed Medicines by Pharmacist and Nurse Independent Prescribers.* Available at www.rpsgb.org.uk/pdfs/LEBunlicensedmed.pdf.

FURTHER READING

Department of Health (2006) *Medicines Matters. A Guide to Mechanisms for the Prescribing, Supply and Administration of Medicines.* Available at www.dh.gov.uk/dr_consum_dh/groups/dh_digitalassets/@dh/@en/documents/digitalasset/dh_064326.pdf.

Department of Health, 6 January 2010. *Nurse Prescribing FAQ.* Available at www.dh.gov.uk/en/Healthcare/Medicinespharmacyandindustry/Prescriptions/TheNon-MedicalPrescribingProgramme/Nurseprescribing/DH_4123003.

Department of Health, 12 March 2007. *Supplementary Prescribing FAQ.* Available at www.dh.gov.uk/en/Healthcare/Medicinespharmacyandindustry/Prescriptions/TheNon-MedicalPrescribingProgramme/Supplementaryprescribing/DH_4123034.

Department of Health National Practitioner Programme, DH Core Prescribing Group Publication only available electronically at www.

dh.gov.uk/dr_consum_dh/groups/dh_digitalassets/@dh/@en/
documents/digitalasset/dh_064326.pdf

National Prescribing Centre, updated 21 December 2009. *Non-medical Prescribing Frequently Asked Questions.* Available at hwww.npc.co.uk/prescribers/faq.htm.

Index

Index